FREUD

&

Psychoanalysis

Gethsemani Studies
in Psychological and Religious Anthropology

ERNEST DANIEL CARRERE, O.C.S.O.
Series Editor

has been funded through a generous grant by
RICHARD C. COLTON, JR.

FREUD

&

Psychoanalysis

W. W. MEISSNER, S. J., M. D.

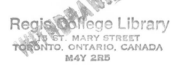
University of Notre Dame Press
Notre Dame, Indiana

Analytic
Table of Contents

Irenaeus of Lyons nearly two millennia earlier: "Irrational . . . are they who await not the time of increase, but . . . being insatiable and ungrateful, unwilling to be at the outset what they have also been created—men subject to passions—go beyond the law of the human race, and before they become men, they wish to be even now like God their creator . . ." (IV.38.4). If it is onerous to be human, the dissociation that plagues our species, as both Freud and Irenaeus suggest, tends toward the pole of spirit. The challenge is to embrace the earth of our humanity.

Thomas Merton pointed out that a common apprehension has Freud declaring that restrictions of conventional morality are injurious because they impede or frustrate sexual desire. "In point of fact," Merton writes in *Contemplation in a World of Action* (p. 36), "this is not what Freud is saying. Freud is deploring a social situation in which man does not learn to love in a full and mature manner insofar as his passions remain in a crude infantile state which keeps him from being fully human, fully able to give himself in love." Freud's point, Merton emphasizes, is that a human being must develop in such a way that one is not overwhelmed by blind forces that can otherwise be integrated into a mature identity: the union of psyche and soma.

Thus, Dr. Meissner's authoritative study, uniting a lucid exposition of the evolution of Freud's thought with a synthesis of contemporary psychoanalytic theory—including the contributions of Margaret Mahler and Erik Erikson, as well as those of Heinz Hartmann, Heinz Kohut, Otto Kernberg, Ronald Fairbairn, Donald Winnicott, and Anna Freud—is the second volume of Gethsemani Studies in Psychological and Religious Anthropology.

Gethsemani Studies is a series of books that explores, through the twin perspectives of psychology and religion, the dynamics and depths of being fully human. An integrated or dialogical perspective is always anticipated in the works; nevertheless, a title favoring the religious standpoint may appear if it bears psychological ramifications, while a title devoted to psychological issues may appear if it is foundational or contributes to the integrated and humanizing dialogue.

This dialogue embraces the entire range of dynamic psychology, from Freud and Jung to Kohut and Lacan, with special predilection, perhaps, for the insights of psychoanalytic object relations theory, while the work of Kernberg, Spotnitz, and Searles, to name only three, offers the promise of equal enrichment.

Gethsemani Studies would have remained an impossibility without the presence of Dick Colton. Dick recognized in the earliest, most speculative discussions that the series represented a worthy project. His dedicated interest cut through the hesitation that impedes new endeavors, inspiring the involvement of all, while his generous grant underwriting the series enabled Notre Dame and the Abbey of Gethsemani to work concretely toward its realization.

Jeff Gainey of the University of Notre Dame Press immediately perceived the potential of such a series and has labored as a wonderful colleague to realize its possibilities. Jim Langford, then press director and now director emeritus, has been an essential collaborator, sagely contributing insights from his rich publishing experience. Barbara Hanrahan, Director of the University of Notre Dame Press, has brought a delightful and cogent presence to our deliberations. The superb staff of the press has continued to be a marvelous joy throughout our preparations. Wendy McMillen deserves special thanks for her superlative book designs, as does Margaret Gloster for the magnificent covers she has created for the series. Fr. Timothy Kelly, Abbot of Gethsemani, has made it possible for me to assume the full-time burdens and joys that being editor imparts.

Richard and Janita Rawls, as wonderful friends and wise colleagues, were primary consultants at the threshold of the series who provided substantial and reliable counsel.

Brigitte Manteuffel has been an indispensable collaborator in corroborating quotations and citations. For this volume, she generously rerouted a trip in order to convey two weighty and hard-to-find books to our corner of Kentucky, then volunteered to track down an elusive journal that wasn't accessible through available resources. In addition, Brian Barlow, Alexandra Moore, and Suzie Sherrill have all contributed to the project.

Introduction

The present work will present a relatively comprehensive and synthetic statement of the current state of psychoanalytic theory. The importance of that enterprise should not be underestimated for the potential student of general psychiatry. Psychoanalysis has existed since the turn of the century, and in that four score and more of years, it has established itself as a fundamental discipline within psychiatry. The science of psychoanalysis is the bedrock of psychodynamic understanding, and it forms the fundamental theoretical frame of reference for a variety of forms of therapeutic intervention, embracing not only the psychoanalytic technique itself but various forms of psychoanalytically oriented psychotherapy and related forms of therapy in which psychodynamic concepts are employed. A case can even be made that more recent theoretical approaches using modifications of systems theory embody many of the suppositions of psychoanalytic theory, for example, family dynamics and the operations of family emotional systems. Consequently, an informed and clear understanding of the fundamental facets of psychoanalytic theory and orientation are essential for the student's grasp of a large and significant segment of current psychiatric thinking.

This dimension of the psychoanalytic enterprise maintains its validity even in the face of the often stringent criticisms made of psychoanalytic formulations on scientific grounds. In fact, psychoanalytic

theory does not represent an amalgamation of dogmatic pronouncements; it stakes its claim to validity on scientific grounds. It is
therefore open to all the vicissitudes of revision, reconsideration, and
questioning in the light of new and pertinent data and has in fact
demonstrated throughout its long history a continual evolution and
modification of its concepts. The basic question concerns whether
psychoanalysis can be regarded as a science and, if so, what kind? The
criticisms launched against psychoanalysis from the side of positivistic philosophy, in which the model of science is based on an analysis
of physical sciences, have found considerable fault with the methodology and the theoretical formulations proposed by psychoanalysis.
More recent reflections on this issue, however, have revised earlier
pronouncements and have tended to see the more puristic and positivistic criteria for authentic science as being excessively rigid and
narrow. Further study seems to suggest that even the physical sciences
have difficulty in adhering to the positivistic criteria. Notions of what
in fact is required for valid scientific work have evolved more in the direction of accepting the possibility of subjective components. It is in
this realm of mixed methodology that psychoanalysis flourishes.

Many psychoanalytic theorists, largely influenced by models of
physical science, have insisted that psychoanalysis is essentially an empirical observational science; that is, that it is based on observable scientific data. The difficulties in such an approach have led other theorists to completely abandon an objective "scientific" rationale and to
opt for a linguistic or hermeneutic approach that envisions psychoanalysis as a fundamentally humanistic discipline that concerns itself
with meanings and the relationships of meaning, rather than with observable events and causes. This latter approach, however, seems to
throw the baby out with the bathwater. Such polarization seems to
move toward another rather rigid and narrow position that would
deny psychoanalysis any scientific validity.

The approach on which the present account is based seeks a middle
ground, one that of itself has its complexities and difficulties, but one
that seems somehow closer to the nature of psychoanalytic work and
the psychoanalytic inquiry. It presumes that psychoanalysis is indeed a
valid science, but it is a science of a very particular sort, one that seeks
and embraces the inner psychic life of human beings, an inner life that
is impregnated with meaning and purpose, that is governed by signifi-

cance and intentionality, but at the same time both reflects and is influenced by a variety of degrees and forms of causality.

One of the difficulties in presenting such a synthetic account is that it must draw its material from more than three-quarters of a century of thinking and theoretical development. Although a variety of approaches might be adopted to the diversity of such material, the author has opted to organize this material along two distinguishable lines that at times are in conjunction, but at other times are more or less out of phase. The one line is that of historical sequence, and the second line of organization is conceptual. Consequently, although the material has an implicit historical reference that spans the earliest beginnings of Freud's psychoanalytic thinking from even before 1900 until some of the most recent developments of object relations theory and self-psychology, there are numerous points in this accounting in which the historical framework is overridden by the demands of conceptual integration. The reader, therefore, will have to keep one eye on the historical dimension, while keeping a second eye on the patterns of conceptual integration. The author will attempt to be explicit about these shifts in orientation as the material develops.

There are, of course, significant risks in approaching material of this kind from such a perspective. To begin with, there is a considerable degree of compression and collapsing of material from a variety of sources. Although such an approach lends a degree of conceptual clarity, it runs a risk of oversimplification and tends to generate an account that is excessively abstract or removed from its roots in clinical data. It is not always possible to articulate the connection of theoretical formulations with their underlying clinical substratum, so that the reader must constantly bear in mind that the clinical basis lies behind the specific formulations and that, unless one is able to bring one's understanding of the theory to the clinical situation and apply it there in a meaningful way, the theory will have lost its significance and will have become a relatively empty exercise in abstraction.

An additional risk that a synthetic and general account such as this might run is that it is in danger of giving the impression that the theory has somehow arrived at a state of static consistency and that the propositions involved are matters of general and unquestioned acceptance. The fact is far removed from such a picture. Throughout its history, even in the hands of Freud himself, psychoanalytic understanding has

Freud and His Scientific *Project*

PSYCHOANALYSIS WAS the child of Freud's genius. He put his stamp on it from the very beginning, and it can be fairly said that, although the science of psychoanalysis has advanced far beyond Freud's wildest dreams, his influence is still strong and pervasive. In understanding the origins of psychoanalytic thinking, it is useful to keep in mind that Freud himself was an outstanding product of the scientific training and thinking of his era.

Scientific Orientation

Freud was a convinced empirical scientist whose early training in medicine and neurology had been carried out at the most progressive scientific centers of his time. He shared the conviction of most of the scientists of his day that scientific law and order and the systematic study of physical and neurological processes would ultimately yield an understanding of the apparent chaos of mental processes. When he began his study of hysteria, he believed that brain physiology was the definitive scientific approach and that it alone would yield a truly scientific understanding of this entity.

With time and with his own increasing clinical experience, Freud was forced to modify that basic scientific credo, but it is significant

foundations for his own thinking and provided the substratum on
which the superstructure of psychoanalysis was raised. From the historical vantage point, one can look back and see the tremendous influence that the ideas of the *Project* had on the development of Freud's
thought, even into the later stages of his career. At those points in his
thinking in which Freud was dealing with the economic and energic
aspects of psychic functioning, the influence of the *Project* is apparent,
and it is for this reason a document of supreme importance.

The influence of the *Project*, then, permeates Freud's thinking and
writing on many levels. During the period of his struggles with the
ideas in the *Project*, he was working with Breuer on the problem of
hysteria. In 1893, they published a "Preliminary Communication" in
which they sketched some of their ideas about the nature of hysteria.
Finally, they published *Studies on Hysteria* in 1895. In both the "Preliminary Communication" and the *Studies*, the influence of the ideas
of the *Project* can be seen, particularly in the notions of cerebral excitation and of discharge of affect. Later, in 1900, in the famous seventh
chapter of Freud's *The Interpretation of Dreams*, the model of the mind
he proposed there has direct links to the concepts of mental functioning formulated in the *Project*. Still later, in his development of a theory
of sexuality and in his elaboration of an instinct theory, even as late as
1920 in *Beyond the Pleasure Principle*, the influence of the *Project* is explicit and identifiable. Also, it is now clear that many of the formulations that Freud reached in the writing of the *Project* were revived and
found their way into his thinking, once again, in the later development
of an ego theory.

Consequently, the *Project* must be seen as an extremely important
and seminal work. If it brought Freud's neurological period to a bril-
liant close, it also opened the way to the broad vistas of psychoanalysis
and, in extremely important and significant ways, determined the
shape that psychoanalytic principles were to take. Freud states his
intention from the very beginning: "The intention is to furnish a psychology that shall be a natural science: that is, to represent psychical
processes as quantitatively determinant states of specifiable material
particles, thus making those processes perspicuous and free from contradiction" (1 *SE* 295).

The *Project* was an ambitious attempt to be as scientific in the
19th-century sense of Helmholtz as possible. Freud based his thinking

on two principal theorems. The first was a quantitative conception of neural activity that he referred to as Q. Q was a quantity of neural excitation that could be transmitted from cell to cell in the nervous system and from neural system to neural system. The second principal theorem was the neuron doctrine, according to which the nervous system was composed of distinct and similarly constructed neurons that were separated from each other yet in contact with one another through "contact barriers" (synapses).

Freud postulated that there were at least two systems of neurons, which had different characteristics that affected psychological functions. The ϕ-system of neurons consisted of permeable elements whose function was to transmit Q to other neuronal systems without any significant alterations of the ϕ-neurons themselves. The ψ-neurons were, by way of contrast, impermeable; that is, their function was not the transmission of Q but, rather, the reception of Q and the storing of it in such a way as to change the neuron and build up a level of internal charge. Freud saw these combined properties of the respective neuronal systems as explaining one of the peculiarities of the neural system, namely, the capacity for retaining and storing excitations and yet, at the same time, remaining capable of receiving further excitatory input.

Freud described one of the fundamental principles of the operation of the nervous system as the "principle of neuronic inertia." According to this principle, neurons tend to divest themselves of Q, the quantity of excitation. This property, by which the nervous system tended to keep itself free from excitation, led to the process of discharge as one of the primary functions of neuronal systems. Freud called this the "constancy principle," more familiarly known as homeostasis. In 1893, Freud formulated the principle in these words: "If a person experiences a psychical impression, something in his nervous system which we will for the moment call the sum of excitation is increased. Now in every individual there exists a tendency to diminish this sum of excitation once more, in order to preserve his health" (3 *SE* 36). The principle of constancy serves as the economic foundation stone for Freud's instinctual theory (Table 1).

Freud envisioned excitation not as arising spontaneously in the nervous system but, rather, as being put into it from the outside. Q was delivered to the nervous system from two sources. The first was

Table 1.   Energic Principles Based on the *Project*

Entropy	Tendency for energy in any physical system to flow from a region of high energy to regions of lower energy. Tendency of system toward homogeneity. Tendency of system to spontaneously diminish the amount of energy available for work.
Conservation	The sum of forces (energy) in any isolated (closed) system remains constant.
Neuronic inertia	Neurons tend to divest themselves of quantities of excitation. Application of entropy and conservation to neuronal activity.
Constancy	The nervous system tends to maintain itself in a state of constant tension or level of excitation. Return to a level of constant excitation is achieved by a tendency to immediate energic discharge (through the path of least resistance).
Nirvana	The dominant tendency to reduce, keep constant, or remove the internal psychic tension due to the excitation of stimuli. The tendency to reduce the level of excitation to a minimum. Extension of constancy principle. Expressed in pleasure principle, ultimately in death instinct.
Pleasure-Unpleasure	Tendency of mental apparatus to seek pleasure and avoid unpleasure. Unpleasure is due to the increase of tension or level of excitation, while pleasure is due to the release of tension or discharge of excitation. The pleasure principle thus follows the economic requirements of constancy.

external reality, which excited the sensory organs by way of external physical excitation. The second was from the body itself, which provided endogenous stimuli that impinged on the mental apparatus and called equally for discharge. These endogenous stimuli were related to the major needs of the body, including hunger, respiration, and sexuality. Thus, at the root of his thinking, Freud explicitly stated a theory of the nervous system as passively responsive to external sources of stimulation and motivated in terms of drive or tension reduction.

His view of the perceptual process was decidedly Helmholtzian; that is, reality consisted of nothing but material masses in motion, and the roots of the perceptual process lay in the physical excitation of neural elements. Freud was also careful, however, not to leave his system exposed to the destructive impact of excessive excitation. He also postulated that excitation in the system was directly proportional to the amount of stimulation. When sums of excitation met the sensory apparatus, they were broken up into portions of stimulation. This provided a preliminary threshold below which the quantities of excitation were barred from affecting the neuronal system. Consequently, the effectiveness of minor stimuli was minimized, and the system was restrictively responsible to more or less medium quantities of excitation. Freud later referred to this threshold as a stimulus-barrier, the primitive analogue of defense.

After excitation had penetrated to the ϕ-system of permeable neurons, the qualitative characteristics of the stimuli were conveyed unhindered through the ϕ-system to the level of the ψ-system of impermeable neurons. Excitation was again processed in the ψ-system and transmitted to the ω-system, which was composed of perceptual neurons, where the functions of consciousness were carried out. The ψ-nucleus was connected with those paths through which the endogenous quantities of excitation were derived. Endogenous stimuli were presumed to be intercellular in nature. As the ψ-neurons filled with quantities of Q, there resulted an effort to discharge the quantity. The discharge was then effected through motor systems, autonomic discharge, and other effector mechanisms. The problem of how quantitative variation in excitation would give rise to the experience of quality reflected the underlying mind-body problem. The physical reductionism of the Helmholtz view did not admit qualities originating in external reality. Freud solved this difficulty by appealing to the special system of perceptual neurons whose excitation gave rise to the experience of different qualities in the form of conscious sensations (ω).

With regard to the quantities of Q impinging on the neural systems, Freud did not differentiate between the energy from the outside and that from within the organism except in one important detail. The critical difference was that the organism can withdraw itself from external stimuli, but it cannot withdraw itself from the effects of endogenous stimuli. His theory of inner motivation consequently was based on a concept of drive energy and included a notion of discharge and reduction of energic inputs (Figure 1).

Freud then added that the success the nervous system experienced in discharging tension was equivalent to pleasure, just as pain was

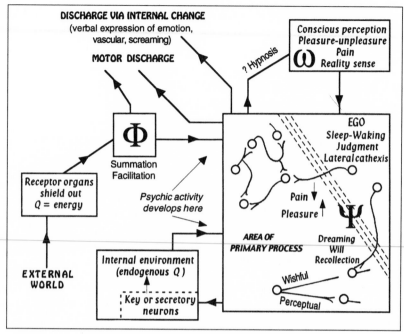

Figure 1.   Summary diagram of the theories in Freud's *Project for a Scientific Psychology*

related to the building up of excessive nervous excitation. Because discharge of excitation was the primary function of the neuronal system, the system was envisioned as ordered to the achieving of pleasure through discharge of excitation and, correspondingly, to the avoidance of pain. Thus, the principle of constancy can be seen to underlie the basic presumptions of Freud's instinctual theory and its relationship to the pleasure principle. The principle of constancy, further, has its roots in the principle of conservation of energy as proposed by Mayer and Helmholtz, according to which the sum of forces remains constant in every closed physical system. The principle also relates to Herbart's hypothesis that mental processes tend to strive for equilibrium—a notion similar to Cannon's concept of homeostasis.

On the basis of these slender postulates, Freud elaborated a complex and ingenious account of mental functions. He was unable, however, to provide a satisfactory account of either defense or consciousness. In both cases he became embroiled in a continuing regress in which he seemed unable to stop. Despite a variety of ingenious feedback loops that he built into the system—Freud was many decades ahead of his time in envisioning informational servomechanisms— Freud was unable to complete the functioning of his system without violating the demands of his mechanical principles. He thus introduced into his system a major concession to vitalism, an observing ego. This observing ego was able to see danger for the mobilization of defenses and was able to sense the indication of quality in conscious experiences. The ego remained as a sort of primary "willer" and ultimate "knower"—a personal center within the theory that could not be reduced to the physicalistic terms of Freud's Helmholtzian postulates and that consequently enjoyed a significant degree of autonomy.

Although the usefulness of these energic postulates is generally recognized to the extent that they provided a useful heuristic basis for the development of Freud's early ideas and for the development of further psychoanalytic ideas, in the last few years these energic concepts have come under stringent methodological criticism. Freud's hypothetical psychic energy was assumed to be at work in the mental apparatus as the motivating force of mental operations, but it had no specified relationship to physical energies operating in the brain. Psychic energy is derived from instinctual drives and is subsequently modified and guided by psychic structures—however, always in the direction of discharge, whether directly or indirectly. The patterns of such discharge are governed by the economic principles already discussed. Nonetheless, Freud's idea that symptoms reflect such indirect patterns of discharge of quantities of energies, which without the presence of neurotic conflict would have been more immediately and freely discharged, was a fundamental and even revolutionary concept.

The most stringent forms of criticism of the notion of psychic energy propose that it fails to meet the most minimal criteria of accepted scientific methodology. Specifically, it is internally contradictory and lacks consistency; it presents a logically closed system that misinterprets metaphor as fact; it involves tautological renaming of observable psychological phenomena in energic terms, which masquerades as explanation; it is unable to explain all the relevant data; it tends to lead to a false sense of explanation, particularly to the extent that it offers pseudoexplanations that are inconsistent with current knowledge of neurophysiology; and, finally, it promotes a form of mind-body dualism that prevents integration of psychoanalytic concepts with other related sciences. Thus, it tends to serve as a substitute for other forms of explanation (for example, neurophysiological) and becomes a barrier rather than a bridge between psychoanalysis and physiology.

Other more specific criticisms attack the concept of psychic energy. Such energy is essentially immeasurable so that, in effect, one is unable to find ways to specifically test quantitative assumptions. This circumstance leaves psychoanalysts more or less in the position of providing descriptions that tend to be taken as explanations. Moreover, the imposition of the concept of psychic energy makes it difficult if not impossible to understand the connection between such energies and the physical energies known to be operating in neurological structures. Consequently, the laws of transformation from one to the other remain unspecified and unknowable. This situation also tends to make it difficult to generate testable hypotheses on the basis of psychoanalytic concepts that might be evaluated by other nonanalytic methodologies.

Another difficulty in this area arises in connection with such qualitatively different forms of psychic energy as libidinal energies, aggressive energies, various degrees of neutralized energies, bound energies, and fused energies. The difficulty here has not so much to do with the varying manifestation of energies in different forms but, rather, with the idea that the differences are inherent in the energies themselves. At one time, physiologists believed that there were specific nerve energies that accounted for the differences in sensory perceptual experience; for example, that different sensory modalities, such as the auditory or visual system, operated on the basis of distinguishable forms of nervous energy specific to each modality. More recent neurophysiology of the nerve impulse, however, indicates that there is no inherent differentiation on the level of neuronal energies and that the differences have to do rather with the central termination and organization of neuronal systems and the patterns of stimulus input. On this particular point, the disparity between the hypothesis of psychic energy and more contemporary views of the functioning of the nervous system seems quite apparent.

Despite these criticisms and difficulties, there still is a substantial number of analytic theorists unwilling to abandon the energic hypothesis. For example, they would argue that the attempt to integrate psychoanalytic findings with the discoveries and concepts of other related scientific fields may be premature. Freud's attempt to do this in the *Project* faltered because too little was known of brain physiology at the time to be useful in explaining his psychological observations. Consequently, he had to develop a rough working hypothesis of some sort of energy characterized by properties that were theoretically useful to him in developing his own ideas, leaving for the future the refinement of this hypothetical notion and its integration with other branches of science.

Despite the tremendous advance in the understanding of neuro-physiology today, it remains questionable whether sufficient understanding of the function of the nervous system has been gained to allow the recasting of energic and structural hypotheses of psychoanalysis in terms of these concepts. Consequently, such theorists argue that the best approach to these problems is to continue to elaborate psycho-analytic theory in whatever way seems to be most useful clinically, without becoming concerned over its relation to or potential integration with data, observations, and theories from other related scientific fields. Further, the inability to measure quantitative dimensions continues to present a problem, but it is not a problem that is foreign to other scientific methods. Psychoanalysis shares such difficulties in quantification with certain of the biological sciences. Moreover, it is characteristic of the early development of many sciences to use relatively primitive forms of quantitative techniques. The difficulty in psychoanalysis is even more marked and understandable in view of the extraordinary complexity of variables, many of which are loosely defined and not specifically interrelated.

One of the difficulties inherent in the discussion of psychic energy is that, because of the original mode in which Freud expressed his economic views, the economic hypothesis has become overidentified with the hypothesis of psychic energy. There is little doubt that psychoanalytic theory cannot do without a principle of economics. It would be impossible to express or understand matters of quantitative variation, degrees of intensity, levels and intensity of motivation, or to explain how individual subjects are able to make choices among conflicting motivations and goals to bring about the resolution of conflict—or for that matter to explain the whole range of affective, motivational, and structural concepts that form the backbone of psychoanalytic understanding—without invoking the very concepts and issues of quantity and intensity that led Freud from the very beginning to postulate an economic point of view.

What remains questionable, however, and what has essentially been the target of the sternest criticisms has been the hypothetical construct of psychic energy. Whether psychoanalysis can sustain a principle of economics without the energic encumbrances derived from late 19th-century physics and physiology remains a point to be argued and discussed. Many theorists have argued that the theoretical utility of an energy-force model has long been outlived and that the contemporary framework of scientific thinking calls much more for an informational-processing model of psychic functioning. The point to be emphasized in the present context is that such a model remains to be adequately developed as a substitute for the theoretical implications of Freud's earlier energic views and that such a model cannot take its potential role in the complexities of psychoanalytic theory without embodying basic economic principles and an economic point of view. Informational and process concepts are no less inherently economic than their energic predecessors. Ultimately, psychoanalysis may have to find a way to conceptually integrate both energic and informational approaches.

TWO

Beginnings
of Psychoanalysis

In the decade extending from 1887 to 1897, the period in which Freud began to seriously study the disturbances of his hysterical patients, the beginnings of psychoanalysis can be said to have taken root. These slender beginnings had a three-fold aspect: the emergence of psychoanalysis as a method of investigation, as a therapeutic technique, and as a body of scientific knowledge based on an increasing fund of information and basic theoretical propositions. These early researches flowed out of Freud's initial collaboration with Joseph Breuer and then, increasingly, out of his own independent investigations and theoretical developments.

The Case of Anna O.

Breuer was an older physician, a distinguished and established practitioner in the Viennese community. Knowing Freud's interests in hysterical pathology, Breuer told him about the unusual case of a woman he had treated for about a year and a half—from December 1880 to June 1882. This was the famous case of Fräulein Anna O., which proved to be one of the important stimuli in the development of psychoanalysis.

Anna O. was, in reality, Bertha Pappenheim, who later became quite famous as a founder of the social work movement. At the time she began to see Breuer, she was an intelligent and strong-minded woman of about twenty-one years of age who had developed a number of hysterical symptoms in connection with the illness and death of her father. These symptoms included paralysis of the limbs, contractures, anesthesias, visual disturbances, disturbances of speech, anorexia, and a distressing nervous cough. Her illness was also characterized by two distinct phases of consciousness; one was relatively normal, but in the other she seemed to assume a second and more pathological personality. These latter states were called absences. The transition between these two states seemed to be brought about by a form of autohypnosis. Breuer became able to manipulate the transition between these two states by placing her in a hypnotic state.

Very fond of and very close to her father, Anna had shared with her mother the duties of nursing him on his deathbed. During her altered states of consciousness, Anna was able to recall the vivid fantasies and intense emotions she had experienced while caring for her father. It was with considerable amazement, both to the patient and to Breuer, that when she was able to recall, with the associated expression of affect, the scenes or circumstances under which her symptoms had arisen, the symptoms could be made to disappear. Anna vividly described this process as the "talking cure" and as "chimney sweeping."

Once the connection between talking through the circumstances of the symptoms and the disappearance of the symptoms themselves had been established, Anna proceeded to deal with each of her many symptoms, one after another. She was able to recall that on one occasion, when her mother had been absent, she had been sitting at her father's bedside and had had a fantasy or daydream in which she imagined that a snake was crawling toward her father and was going to bite him. She struggled forward to try to ward off the snake, but her arm, which had been draped over the back of the chair, had gone to sleep. She was unable to move it. The paralysis remained, and she was unable to move the arm until she was able to recall this scene under hypnosis. It is easy to see how this kind of material must have made a profound impression on Freud. It provided a convincing demonstration of the power of unconscious memories and of suppressed affects in the production of hysterical symptoms.

In the course of the somewhat lengthy treatment, Breuer had become increasingly preoccupied with his fascinating and unusual patient and, consequently, spent more and more time with her. In the meanwhile, his wife had grown increasingly jealous and resentful. As soon as Breuer began to realize this, the sexual connotations of it frightened him, and he abruptly terminated the treatment. Only a few hours later, however, he was recalled urgently to Anna's bedside. She had never alluded to the forbidden topic of sex during the course of her treatment, but she was now experiencing hysterical childbirth. The phantom pregnancy was the logical termination of the sexual feelings she had developed toward Breuer in response to his therapeutic efforts. He had been quite unaware of this development, and the experience was quite unnerving. He was able to calm Anna down by hypnotizing her, but then he left the house in a cold sweat and immediately set out with his wife for Venice on a second honeymoon.

According to a version that comes from Freud through Ernest Jones, the patient was far from cured and had later to be hospitalized after Breuer's departure. It seems ironical that the prototype of a cathartic cure was, in fact, far from successful. Nevertheless, the case of Anna O. provided an important starting point and a crucial juncture in the development of psychoanalysis.

Studies on Hysteria

The collaboration with Breuer brought about the publication of their "Preliminary Communication" in 1893. This was a first step in the direction of psychoanalysis. Essentially, Freud and Breuer extended Charcot's concept of traumatic hysteria to a general doctrine of hysteria. Hysterical symptoms were related to determined psychic traumata, sometimes clearly and directly but also sometimes in a symbolic disguise. The observations based on these later cases establish a connection between the pathogenesis of common hysteria and that of traumatic neurosis; in both cases the trauma is not followed by sufficient reaction and is thus kept out of consciousness.

The authors observe that the individual hysterical symptoms seem to disappear immediately when the event that provoked them was clearly brought to life, with the patient describing the event in great detail and putting the accompanying affect into words. The fading of a memory or the loss of its associated affect depends on various factors, including whether or not there has been an energetic reaction to the event that provoked the affect. Thus, memories can be regarded as traumata that have not been sufficiently abreacted. The authors note that the splitting of consciousness that is so striking in the classical cases of hysteria as "double consciousness" is present to at least a rudimentary degree in every hysteria. The basis of hysteria is described in the "Preliminary Communication" as a hypnoid state; that is, a state of dissociated consciousness. Psychotherapy was thought to achieve its curative effect on hysterical symptoms by bringing to an end the operative force of the idea that was not sufficiently abreacted in the first instance. It does this by allowing the strangulated affect to find a way of discharge through speech and thus subjects it to an associative correction, introducing it into connection with normal consciousness.

The "Preliminary Communication" created considerable interest, and it was followed in 1895 by *Studies on Hysteria* in which Breuer and Freud reported on their clinical experience in the treatment of hysteria and proposed a theory of hysterical phenomena. Freud's case discussions proved to be extremely significant since they formed the original basis for much of his psychoanalytic thinking. The first case history was that of Emmy von N.

Emmy von N. was a woman of about forty years of age whose treatment Freud undertook in 1889. She suffered from a variety of hysterical complaints, including mild deliria, hallucinations, anesthesia and pain in her leg, and an ovarian neuralgia. Freud had no doubt that her pathology was basically hysterical in nature. She also suffered from psychic symptoms, which included alterations of moods, phobias, and abulias. Freud became quite involved in her case, since her personality interested him, and he devoted a considerable amount of time to her treatment. She could be put into a state of somnambulism with considerable ease. Thus, Freud used hypnosis while also applying, for the first time, the cathartic technique, which Breuer had described to him and which Breuer had applied in the treatment of Anna O.

Freud used the hypnosis primarily for the purpose of providing Emmy von N. with maxims, which she could keep in mind and use to protect herself from relapsing into delirious states. Freud felt that the phobias and abulias in this patient were primarily traumatic in origin. The distressing affects connected with these traumatic experiences had remained unresolved. The lively activity of her memory brought these traumas and their accompanying affects little by little into her consciousness and gave rise to the hysterical symptoms.

The second case was Lucy R., whom Freud had treated toward the end of 1892. Referred to Freud by another physician, Lucy R. suffered from a chronically recurrent suppurative rhinitis. At the time, she was also suffering from depression and fatigue and was tormented by subjective sensations of smell, particularly the smell of burnt pudding. Freud was able to determine that this hysterical symptom was related to an event in which the patient's employer had reprimanded her, thus dashing her romantic hopes. The smell was associated with a trauma and persisted in her consciousness as the symbolic representation of the trauma.

Freud concluded from these observations that an experience that had played an important pathogenic role, together with its subsidiary concomitants, was accurately retained in the patient's memory, even when it seemed to be forgotten and the patient was unable to voluntarily recall it to mind. He postulated that as an essential condition for the development of hysteria an idea must be repressed from consciousness and excluded from any modification by association with other ideas. At this early stage, Freud felt that the repression was intentional and that it served as the basis for the conversion of a sum of neural excitation. This sum of excitation, when it was cut off from the more normal paths of psychic association, would find its way all the more easily along a deviant path that led to somatic innervation. The basis for such repression, he argued, must be a feeling of unpleasure that derived from the incompatibility between the idea to be repressed and the dominant mass of ideas that constituted the ego.

Moreover, as one symptom was removed, another would develop to take its place. The illness could be acquired even by a person of sound heredity as the result of the appropriate traumatic experiences. It should be noted that this view was quite different from the view proposed by Breuer, which ascribed the origin of hysteria to hypnoid states. The actual traumatic moment, in Freud's view, was the one in which the incompatibility of ideas forces itself on the ego and in which the ego decides on repudiation of the incompatible idea. This reaction brings into being a nucleus for the crystallization of a psychic group that is somehow divorced from the ego. This process resulted in a splitting of consciousness that was characteristic of acquired hysteria. The therapeutic process consisted in compelling this split-off psychical group to unite once more with the main mass of conscious ego ideas.

The case of Katharina is particularly interesting since it is probably one of the shortest cases of psychoanalytic treatment on record. Katharina was an employee at a mountain resort that Freud visited. She sought Freud out to implore his help with symptoms of anxiety that had first appeared about two years earlier. In the course of a few conversations, Katharina came to realize that her father had been making sexual advances to her and that he had also been sexually involved with her cousin. Freud related her anxiety to the sexual stimulation, which she had put out of her conscious awareness. He thus fitted the case into the schematic picture of an acquired hysteria. Katharina's anxiety was hysterical—that is, it was a reproduction of an anxiety that had appeared in the first instance in connection with earlier and even infantile sexual traumas.

In every case of hysteria based on sexual traumas, Freud felt that the impressions from the presexual period, which produce little or no effect on the child, can attain a traumatic power at a later date as memories when the girl or married woman begins to acquire an understanding and exposure to sexual life.

Finally, Freud discussed the case of Elizabeth von R., a woman of twenty-four who was afflicted with an impairment of her posture. She was unable to walk except with the upper part of her body bent forward and with some means of support (astasia-abasia). She also described a number of pains and hyperalgesias, which seemed to have a hysterical basis. Freud pointed out that the descriptions of her pain and the character of her pain were quite indefinite and that, if the hyperalgesic skin and muscles of her legs were touched, her face assumed a peculiar expression that seemed more akin to pleasure than to pain.

Freud was quite puzzled by the apparent lack of connection between the events in her history and her actual symptoms. Analysis seemed to point to the conversion of a psychic excitation into a physical pain. The conversion did not seem to take place when the impressions were fresh; rather, it seemed to take place in connection with memories of the impressions. Freud felt that such a course of events was not at all unusual and that it played a regular part in the genesis of hysterical symptoms.

He substantiated this theory by a description of the case of Rosalie H., a woman of twenty-three who had been trained as a singer. She complained that in parts of her range she could not control her voice; she had a feeling of choking and constriction in her throat. The hysterical symptoms were found to be related to a sexual approach that had been made by an uncle of hers and that had badly frightened her. Freud was able to rid her of the hysterical symptom by getting her to reproduce the traumatic experiences and to abreact them.

Out of these cases Freud reconstructed the following sequence of steps in the development of hysteria:

1. The patient had undergone a traumatic experience, by which Freud meant an experience that stirred up intense emotion and excitation, that was intensely painful or disagreeable to the individual.
2. The traumatic experience represented to the patient some idea or ideas that were incompatible with the "dominant mass of ideas constituting the ego."
3. This incompatible idea was intentionally dissociated or repressed from consciousness.
4. The excitation associated with the incompatible idea was converted into somatic pathways and resulted in the hysterical manifestations and symptoms.
5. What is left in consciousness is merely a mnemonic symbol that is only connected with the traumatic event by associative links that are frequently enough disguised links.
6. If the memory of the traumatic experience can be brought into consciousness and if the patient is able to release the strangulated affect associated with it, then the affect is discharged and symptoms disappear.

Freud's Technical Evolution

One of the fascinating aspects of the *Studies on Hysteria* is the evolution in Freud's development of technical approaches to the treatment of cases of hysteria. As a result of his early interest in hypnosis, as well as his exposure to hypnotic techniques, both in Charcot's clinic and later at Nancy, when Freud opened his own practice in 1887, he began to use hypnosis intensely in treating his patients. In the beginning his use of hypnosis was primarily as a means of getting patients to rid themselves of their symptoms by means of hypnotic suggestion. It was quickly obvious, however, that although a patient would respond to hypnotic suggestion and try to treat the symptoms as if they did not exist, the symptoms would nonetheless assert themselves during the patient's waking experience.

Freud found the contradiction and superficiality of this approach, as well as its relative ineffectiveness as a means of treatment, a source of increasing dissatisfaction. By this time, however, he had come under Breuer's influence, and the fascination of the case of Anna O. made him eager to learn what it was that lay at the root of his patients' symptoms. Freud's curiosity was stimulated, and his scientific mind felt the impulse to search out the reasons for these events and to learn their causes. This quality of restless and remorseless inquiry is one that stamps the peculiar quality of Freud's mind—a quality that allowed him to seek out reasons and causes where others might have faltered and retreated. It is this same need to plumb the depths that characterizes the essential nature of psychoanalytic treatment even today and sets it apart to some extent from those psychiatric techniques that seek merely to modify or relieve overt symptoms.

By 1889, then, Freud was sufficiently intrigued by Breuer's cathartic method to attempt to use it in conjunction with hypnotic techniques as a means of retracing the histories of neurotic symptoms. In his early efforts, he stayed quite close to the notion of the traumatic origins of hysterical symptoms. Consequently, the goal of treatment was restricted to a removal of symptoms through the recovery and verbalization of the suppressed feelings with which symptoms were associated. This procedure has since been described as "abreaction."

Once again, however, as in the case of hypnotic suggestion, Freud was somewhat dissatisfied with the results of this treatment approach. The beneficial effects of the hypnotic treatment seemed to be transitory; they tended to last, or seemed effective, only as long as the patient remained in contact with the physician. Freud suspected that the alleviation of symptoms was in fact dependent in some manner on the personal relationship between the patient and the physician.

Freud had begun to feel that inhibited sexuality may have had a role to play in the production of the patient's symptoms. Freud's suspicion of a sexual aspect in the treatment of such patients was amply confirmed one day when a female patient awoke from a hypnotic sleep and suddenly threw her arms around his neck. Freud suddenly found himself in the same position that Breuer had found himself in during his earlier treatment of Anna O. Perhaps bolstered by Breuer's experience and apparently able to learn from it, Freud did not panic or retreat in the face of this sexual advance. Rather, the peculiar observant quality of his mind was able to disengage itself sufficiently so that this phenomenon could be treated as a scientific observation.

From this point on, Freud began to understand that the therapeutic effectiveness of the patient-physician relationship, which had seemed so mystifying and problematical to him until this time, could be attributed in fact to its erotic basis. These observations were to become the basis of the theory of transference that he would later develop into an explicit theory of treatment. In any event, these experiences reinforced his dissatisfaction with hypnotic techniques. He became aware that hypnosis was masking and concealing a number of important manifestations that seemed to be related to the process of cure or, in some cases, to the failure of the patient to achieve a definitive resolution of the neurosis. Later, his dissatisfaction with hypnosis would become more specific in that he could see that the continued use of hypnosis precluded the investigation of transference and resistance phenomena.

In fact, the decision to shift from the use of Breuer's cathartic method was based on somewhat less sophisticated and mundane considerations. Freud felt uncomfortable with the hypnotic technique because it increasingly became apparent that the hypnotic method was in part successful because of the patient's emotional attachment to the doctor. Often in his experience the patient would recall traumatic experiences or feelings at the doctor's request and frequently would appear to recover from the illness, apparently to please the doctor. Freud felt that a cure that did not involve some understanding on the part of the patient of the origins and significance of the symptoms and that did not base itself on some more scientific approach to the problem could not be expected to be a reliable cure; at best it was a temporary expedient.

There were other reasons for abandoning the cathartic method. Freud had discovered that many of the patients he treated in his pri-

vate practice were in fact refractory to hypnosis. Only gradually did
he come to recognize that what seemed to be his inability to hypnotize
a patient might often enough be due to a patient's reluctance to re-
member traumatic events. He was able later to identify this reluctance as resistance. The vagaries of the hypnotic method did not satisfy Freud, and he felt it necessary to develop an approach to treatment
that could be usefully applied regardless of whether the patient was
hypnotizable or not. Consequently, although Freud continued to use
the hypnotic technique as a basic approach to the treatment of hysteria, he began to experiment with it and gradually succeeded in modifying the technique.

"Concentration" Method

One of the patients whom Freud found to be refractory to the hypnotic technique was Elizabeth von R. For the first time, in this case,
Freud decided to abandon hypnosis as his primary therapeutic tool.
He based his decision to alter his technique in this instance on the observation of Bernheim that, although certain experiences appeared to
be forgotten, they could be recalled under hypnosis and then subsequently recalled consciously if the physician were to ask the patient
leading questions to urge the production of these critical memories.
Freud thus evolved his method of concentration.

The patient was asked to lie down on a couch and to close her
eyes. She was then instructed to concentrate on a particular symptom and to recall the memories associated with it. The method was
substantially a modification of the technique of hypnotic suggestion.
Freud would press his hand on the patient's forehead and urge her
to recall the unavailable memories. Freud's graphic descriptions of this
technique carry with them the unavoidable impression that he was
struggling against a force he sensed in the patient and against which he
found himself battling, as though in a hand-to-hand combat. He came
slowly, by dint of this laborious experience, to realize that the isolation
of certain memory contents was a matter of the operation of mental
forces that generated considerable power and that operated to keep the
complex of pathogenic ideas separate from the mass of conscious ideation. This substantially provided him both with the empirical notion
of resistance and with the basic metapsychological perspective of the
mind as operating in terms of psychic forces.

Technique of Free Association

The material presented in such graphic detail in *Studies on Hysteria* reflects in a dramatic way the evolution of Freud's technique in the direction of his definitive approach to psychoanalysis. What is rehearsed there is the progression from the more hypnotically oriented and derived techniques of the original cathartic method introduced by Breuer to what was to become the staple of psychoanalytic technique, the method of free association. This evolution took place only gradually, and with a slowly dawning realization in the mind of Freud, over at least a three-year period from 1892 until 1895.

He became increasingly convinced by the late 1890s that the process of urging, pressing, questioning, and trying to defeat the resistance offered by the patient—all of which were part and parcel of the "concentration" method—rather than facilitating the overcoming of the patient's resistances actually interfered with the free flow of the patient's thoughts. Piece by piece, Freud thus gave up the elements of the concentration method. Through this progressive evolution, the basic rule of psychoanalysis—free association—was focused and articulated. Gradually, Freud surrendered his technique of forehead pressure, as well as the requirement that patients close their eyes while lying on the couch. The only remnant of this earlier procedure persisting in the practice of psychoanalysis is the use of the couch. The emergence of the central rule of psychoanalysis was the essential product of Freud's evolution.

The evolution of Freud's technique continued to progress until the associative technique had been perfected. The modification of technique that had taken its origin in the case of Elizabeth von R. continued on in this period, with an increasing reliance on the patient's capacity to freely manifest the mental content without suggestive interference on the part of the therapist. By the end of the century, Freud had more or less established his associative technique. In the *Interpretation of Dreams*, he describes it in the following terms:

> This [technique] involves some psychological preparation of the patient. We must aim at bringing about two changes in him: an increase in the attention he pays to his own psychical perceptions and the elimination of the criticism by which he normally sifts the thoughts that occur to him. In order that he may be able to con-

centrate his attention on his self-observation it is an advantage for him to lie in a restful attitude and to shut his eyes. It is necessary to insist explicitly on his renouncing all criticism of the thoughts that he perceives. We therefore tell him that the success of the psychoanalysis depends on his noticing and reporting whatever comes into his head and not being misled, for instance, into suppressing an idea because it strikes him as unimportant or irrelevant or because it seems to him meaningless. He must adopt a completely impartial attitude to what occurs to him, since it is precisely his critical attitude which is responsible for his being unable, in the ordinary course of things, to achieve the desired unravelling of his dream or obsessional idea or whatever it may be. [4 *SE* 101]

Only a few years more and the closing of the eyes was also abandoned. Thus, free association became the definitive technique of psychoanalysis. In fact it was the development of this technique that opened the door to the exploration of dreams, which became one of the primary sources of data that bolstered the nascent psychoanalytic point of view.

Theoretical Innovations

The theoretical point of view propounded in *Studies on Hysteria* was relatively complex. The theoretical section of that work was provided by Breuer, but the fascinating aspect of that section is that Breuer's theoretical formulations reveal in a profound manner the influence of Freud's thinking—or at least a basic scientific orientation that profoundly affected both men. This aspect of the theoretical formulations in the *Studies* was not appreciated until Freud's manuscript on the *Project* became available in 1950.

Etiology of Hysteria

Breuer adopted the point of view that hysterical phenomena are not altogether ideogenic; that is, that they were not determined simply by ideas. In fact the phenomena of hysteria may be determined by a variety of causes, some of them brought about by an explicitly psychical mechanism, but others without it. Although the so-called hysterical phenomena are not necessarily caused by ideas alone, their ideogenic aspects are specifically described as hysterical. The contribution of Freud and Breuer was that they focused on the investigation of these ideogenic aspects and discovered some of their psychic origins. Particularly, the concept of neuronal excitation, which was conceived of as subject to processes of hydraulic flow and discharge, was of fundamental importance in the understanding of hysteria, as well as of neurosis in general.

A careful reading of Breuer's theoretical section in *Studies* makes it abundantly clear that what he proposes is a reworking of the ingenious ideas of Freud's *Project*, with a specific application to the explanation of hysterical phenomenon. Breuer describes two extreme conditions of central nervous system excitation; namely, a clear waking state and the state of dreamless sleep. When the brain is performing actual work, greater consumption of energy is required than when it is merely prepared to do work. The phenomenon of spontaneous awakening can take place in conditions of complete quiet and darkness without any external stimulus. This demonstrates that the development of psychic energy is based on the vital processes of the neural elements themselves.

Speech can serve an important discriminating function. It distinguishes between those forms and degrees of the heightening of excitation that are useful for mental activity because they raise the level of free energy of all the cerebral functions uniformly and those forms and degrees that only restrict mental activity to the extent that they only partly increase and partly inhibit these psychic functions in a relatively nonuniform manner. The former processes are described as incitement, whereas the latter are described as excitement. Excitement seeks to discharge itself in more or less violent ways that can be actually pathological. The psychic component of these aspects is composed of a disturbance of the dynamic equilibrium of the nervous system. Thus, acute affects are based on the disturbances of mental equilibrium that accompany such states of increased excitation. Such activated affects level out the increased intensity of excitation by means of motor discharge. If the affect cannot find a pathway or discharge of excitation, then the level of intracerebral excitation is powerfully increased, even as it cannot be used in associative or motor pathways of discharge.

Breuer also provided an explanation of the process of hysterical conversion. The resistances in relatively normal people to the passage of cerebral excitation by way of the vegetative organs corresponds after a fashion to the insulation of electrical lines of conduction. At the point at which they are abnormally weak, they can be broken through when the tension of cerebral excitation is elevated. Thus, the affective excitation can pass over into the peripheral organs. The result is an abnormal expression of emotion based on two causal factors. The first is the high degree of intracerebral excitation, which has not been leveled down either by ideational association or by motor discharge. The second factor was described as an abnormal weakness of the resistances in particular paths of conduction. Thus, the level of intracerebral excitation and that of excitation in the peripheral paths were regarded as reciprocal. The level of intracerebral excitation increased if, and only if, no reflex action was elicited. The level, however, diminishes when it has been transformed into peripheral nervous excitation. Consequently, it followed that there could be no observable effect if the idea that gave rise to it should immediately release an abnormal reflex into which the excitation could flow as soon as it was generated. Under these circumstances hysterical conversion was complete.

The hysterical phenomena, or the so-called abnormal reflexes, show little evidence of ideogenic origins because the idea that gives rise to the reflex discharge is no longer colored with affect and no longer marked out among other ideas and memories in the mental content. The discharge of affect follows the principle of least resistance and thus takes place along the paths whose resistances have already been weakened. Thus, the genesis of hysterical phenomena that are related to trauma finds a perfect analogy in the hysterical conversion of psychic excitation, which originates not simply from external stimuli, nor from the inhibition of normal psychic reflexes, but from an inhibition of the course of association. In all such cases, there must be a convergence of a number of factors before a hysterical symptom can be generated in an individual who has previously been normal. Affective ideas can be excluded from such association in two ways: either through defense or in situations in which the idea cannot be remembered, as for example in hypnotic states.

The basic explanatory concept that Breuer advanced—not originally, it might be noticed, because the concept had previously been a part of the thinking of French psychiatrists, particularly Janet— was the notion of hypnoid states. Such states were thought to resemble the basic condition of dissociation that obtained in hypnosis. Their importance lies in the amnesia that accompanied them and in their power to bring about a condition of splitting of the mind. The spontaneous origin of such states through a process of autohypnosis was identifiable relatively frequently in a number of fully developed hysterics. These states often alternated rapidly with normal waking states. The experience of the autohypnotic state was found to be subjected to a more or less total amnesia when the patient was in the waking state. The hysterical conversion seemed to take place more easily in such autohypnotic states than in waking states, similar to the more facile realization of suggested ideas in states of artificial hypnosis.

Neither the hypnoid state during periods of energetic work nor the unemotional twilight states are pathogenic. The reveries, however, which were filled with emotion and states of fatigue arising from protracted affects, did seem to be pathogenic. The occurrence of such hypnoid states was important in the genesis of hysterical phenomena because they somehow made conversion easier and prevented, by way of the resulting amnesia, the converted ideas from wearing away and losing their intensity.

It must be said that Freud had little sympathy with Breuer's concept of hypnoid states, although at the stage of *Studies on Hysteria*, Freud had not been able to bring himself to reject it. The concept, in fact, did not explain very much. The hypnoid state was appealed to as an explanation for hysterical states, but the occurrence and function of hypnoid states themselves were in no way explained or supported. They were merely postulated. The only explanatory attempt was made in terms of a hereditary disposition to such states. This unproven postulate was one that Freud's intensely scientific attitude could not accept.

Breuer went on to describe the origin of unconscious ideas. Much of what falls under the heading of "mood" comes from ideas that exist and operate beneath the threshold of consciousness. The whole conduct of life is constantly influenced by such unconscious ideas. All intuitive activity is governed by ideas that are to a significant degree subconscious. Only the clearest and most intense ideas are available to self-consciousness, whereas the great mass of current but less intense ideational content remains unconscious. Breuer related the occurrence of pathological phenomena to the persistence of such unconscious ideas. The existence of such ideas, which are inadmissible to conscious awareness, is a source of pathology.

Janet had proposed that there was a particular form of congenital mental weakness that underlies the disposition to hysteria. The position adopted by Breuer and Freud, however, opposed that of Janet and denied that the splitting of consciousness was based on an inherent weakness in patients. Rather, their own hysterical patients seemed to be individuals of high ideals, vivid and strong imaginations, and in many ways quite vigorous personalities. The appearance of weak-mindedness was simply due to the division in their mental activity that resulted in only a portion of their capacity being placed at the disposal of their conscious thought processes. The dissociation and splitting of the mind was in fact due to the coexistence of two heterogeneous trains of ideas. This splitting seemed also to be responsible for the apparent suggestibility of some hysterical patients, because the unconscious split was responsible for a relative poverty and incompleteness of ideational content.

The notion of an innate disposition served Breuer as a basic foundation on which he based the explanation of hypnoid states. He felt that the capacity to acquire hysteria was closely linked to this idiosyncrasy of innate disposition. Thus, a surplus of excitation that was liberated by the nervous system in a state of rest was thought to determine the patient's incapacity to tolerate a monotonous life and boredom, as well as the patient's craving for sensations that would interrupt this monotony. Such a surplus of excitation can also give rise to pathological manifestations in the motor sphere as well as, for example, tic-like movements. Thus, a number of nervous symptoms, including pain and vasomotor phenomena and, perhaps, purely motor epileptic attacks, are not the result of pathogenic ideas but are the direct result of a fundamental abnormality of the nervous system.

Closely related to these symptoms are the ideogenic phenomena, the simple conversion of affective excitation. Such phenomena are forms of purely somatic hysterical symptoms, whereas the idea that is related to them and gives rise to them can be fended off and consequently repressed. The most frequent and intense of these fended-off and converted ideas have a specifically sexual content. The tendency to fend off such sexual ideas is intensified by the fact that, in young un-married women, sensual excitation is accompanied by anxiety, fear, and apprehension of what is unknown and half-suspected. In addition to such sexual hysteria, there are also hysterical states caused by fright; that is, the so-called traumatic hysterias that constitute one of the major forms of hysterical manifestations. Basic to these hysterical states, and a major constituent of them, was the innate disposition that gave rise to the so-called hypnoid state manifested in a tendency to autohypnosis.

The spirit that moves through Freud's treatment of the psycho-therapy of hysteria is quite different from that embodied in Breuer's theoretical treatment. The discussion of the treatment of hysteria in the *Studies* gives one a good sense of the extent to which Freud had moved away in his own thinking from the somewhat restrictive formu-lations of the *Project*. Freud pointed out that each individual hysterical symptom seemed to disappear more or less permanently when the memory of the traumatic event by which it was provoked was brought into conscious awareness along with its accompanying affect. It was necessary that the patient describe such traumatic events in the great-est possible detail and be able to put into verbal expression the affective experience connected with it.

Freud felt that the basic etiology of the acquisition of neurosis had to be located in sexual factors. Different sexual influences oper-ated to produce different pictures of neurotic disorders. Usually the neurotic picture was a mixed one, and the purer forms of either hys-terical or obsessional neurosis were relatively rare. Freud did not re-gard all hysterical symptoms as psychogenic in origin, and he felt that they could not all be effectively treated by a psychotherapeutic proce-dure. In the context of his theory and technique at that time, he found that a significant number of patients could not be hypnotized despite an apparently certain diagnosis of hysteria. In these patients Freud felt that he had to overcome a certain psychic force in the patient, a force that was set in opposition to any attempt to bring the pathogenic idea into consciousness. In the therapy, he experienced himself engaging in sometimes forceful psychic work to overcome this intense counter-force.

The pathogenic idea, however, despite the force of resistance, was always close at hand and could be reached by relatively easily accessible associations. The patient seemed to be able to get rid of such ideas by turning them into words and describing them. Nevertheless, it was Freud's experience that, in cases wherein he was able to surmise the manner in which things were connected and could tell the patient before the patient had actually uncovered it, the therapist could not force anything on the patient about matters in which the patient was essentially ignorant, nor could the therapist influence the product of the analysis by arousing the patient's expectations.

Freud's development of the technique of free association illuminated a number of significant aspects of mental functioning that had never been previously observed. First of all, Freud discovered that the patient's train of memories extended well beyond the traumatic events that were responsible for precipitating the onset of illness. Indeed, he found that his patients were able to produce such memories of childhood experiences, events, and scenes that had long been lost to memory. This fact led Freud to the conclusion that, frequently enough, such memories had been previously inhibited because they involved sexual experiences or other painful incidents in the patient's life that seemed intolerable to hold in memory.

The recollection of such experiences, even in the present, could evoke intense affects of agitation, moral conflict, feelings of self-reproach or remorse, or fear of punishment and guilt. Freud concluded that, because these childhood experiences retained such a vivid quality, they must exert a predisposing influence on the development of psychoneurotic manifestations. This point of view ran substantially counter to the prevailing attitude of the time. Particularly, it ran counter to the point of view expressed by Breuer in his endorsement of hypnoid states as the explanatory basis for hysteria.

Freud, however, did not abandon the congenital point of view, namely, that heredity must be accorded a major role as a predisposing factor to neurosis. In fact, that point of view remains a significant part of the psychoanalytic understanding of neurosis even today. Nevertheless, Freud placed an important emphasis on unfavorable childhood experiences in his explanation of the etiology of psychoneurosis. Essentially, he postulated that hysteria can also be acquired and that it was not simply a congenitally derived condition. Even further, he postulated that emotionally disturbing experiences could play a major role, particularly in the etiology of acquired hysteria, whereas the hereditary factors seemed to be of minor importance. It should be noted that Freud's views in this regard were a substantial and original contribution to the therapy of neurosis and, particularly, to that of hysteria.

Concept of Resistance

The basic question that confronted Freud and Breuer had to do with the mechanism that made the pathogenic memories unconscious. The divergence in their points of view was not simply a matter of theoretical differences. Freud's own thinking underwent a definite transition, and the transition seemed to be based primarily on Freud's own experience in dealing with his patients. In the beginning he and Breuer had agreed that their hysterical patients had suffered from traumatic sexual experiences. These traumatic experiences were not available to conscious recollection. They had also agreed, at least for a time, that the recovery of these forgotten experiences during a hypnotic state resulted in abreaction and the consequent symptomatic improvement.

Breuer's explanation for this state of affairs rested on the concept of the hypnoid state. The hypnoid state was an altered state of consciousness in which part of the mind was split off from the rest of the mind in a state of dissociation. This splitting was a result of the stress of emotional arousal, so that the normal course of emotional reaction and expression was inhibited. Thus, the content of the dissociated part was isolated from associative links with the rest of consciousness, but these links could be reestablished through hypnosis. Breuer felt that the traumatic experiences must have occurred at a time when the patient was in one of these hypnoid states, so that the traumatic experience had been dissociated. To Breuer's mind, then, the therapeutic work consisted merely of reestablishing associative links.

The divergence between Breuer's and Freud's viewpoints was apparent from the beginning of their collaboration. Even in the "Preliminary Communication," they described two kinds of hysteria, dispositional and psychically acquired. The former was based on Breuer's notion of hypnoid states, but the latter, psychically acquired hysteria, was a condition that could only be acquired by the reaction of the personality to external trauma. Essentially, this was Freud's view. Freud's

halfhearted endorsement of Breuer's notion of hypnoid states would
not fade until he had analyzed the cases of Lucy and Elizabeth von R.
It was only in the treatment of Elizabeth that Freud came to a clear-cut
formulation of his notion of defense. He recognized the conflict between her sexual impulses and her moral convictions. The hypnoid hypothesis was insufficient because the sexual thoughts, Freud felt, were
originally conscious and had to be excluded from the patient's consciousness. Thus, the two sides of the conflict seemed to coexist in the
same system of consciousness. Freud moved in the direction of understanding the basic meaning of hysteria in terms of conflict and a need
for defense against repugnant thoughts and wishes.

Freud discovered that his patients were often quite unwilling or unable to recall the traumatic memories. He defined this reluctance of his
patients as resistance. As his clinical experience expanded, he found
that, in the majority of patients he treated, resistance was not a matter
of reluctance to cooperate; that is, the patients willingly engaged in
the treatment process and were willing to obey the fundamental rule
of free association. The patients generally seemed to be well motivated
for treatment, and frequently enough it was particularly the patients
who were most distressed by their symptoms who seemed most ham-
pered in treatment by the presence of resistance. Freud's conclusion
was that resistance was a matter of the operation of active forces in the
mind, of which the patients themselves were often quite unaware, that
maintained the exclusion from consciousness of painful or distressing
material. The active force that worked to exclude particular mental
contents from conscious awareness Freud described as repression, one
of the fundamental ideas of psychoanalytic theory.

Concept of Repression

The concept of repression, together with its related notion of defense, came to be the basic explanation for hysterical phenomena in
Freud's thinking. The notion of repression reflects one of the basic
hypotheses of psychoanalytic theory, namely, the dynamic hypothesis according to which the human mind includes in its operation
basic dynamic forces that can be set in opposition and that serve as the
basic source of powerful motivation and defense. Freud described the
mechanism of repression in the following terms: A traumatic experience or a series of experiences, usually of a sexual nature and often

occurring in childhood, had been "forgotten" or "repressed" because of their painful or disagreeable nature; but the excitation involved in the sexual stimulation was not extinguished, and traces of it persisted in the unconscious in the form of repressed memories. These memories could remain without pathogenic effect until some contemporary event, as for example a disturbing love affair, served to revive them. At this juncture, the strength of the repressive counterforce was diminished, and the patient experienced what Freud termed "the return of the repressed." The original sexual excitement is revived and finds its way by a new path that allows it to manifest itself in the form of a neurotic symptom. Thus, the symptom results from a compromise between the repressed desire and the "dominant mass of ideas constituting the ego." The whole process of repression and the return of the repressed is thus conceived of as conflicting forces; that is, the force of the repressed idea struggling to express itself against the counterforce of the ego seeking to keep the repressed idea out of consciousness.

Freud's development of the notions of repression and resistance were based primarily on his studies of the cases of conversion hysteria. Specifically, in such cases he felt that the impulses that were not allowed access to consciousness were diverted into paths of somatic innervation, thus resulting in such hysterical symptoms as paralysis, blindness, disturbances of sensations, and other manifestations. Despite this early emphasis on conversion hysteria as the prototype of repression, Freud believed that the basic proposition that symptoms were a result of a compromise between a repressed impulse and other repressing forces could be applied to obsessive-compulsive phenomena and even to paranoid ideation. The logical consequence of this hypothesis was that the treatment process during this period focused primarily on enabling the patient to recall the repressed sexual experiences, so that the accompanying excitation could be allowed to find its way into consciousness and thus be discharged along with the revivified and previously dammed-up affect.

The Seduction Hypothesis and the Theory of Infantile Sexuality

There was one additional aspect of psychoanalytic theory that emerged with striking clarity from these early researches into hysteria.

Invariably, when inquiring into the past histories of his hysterical patients, Freud found that the repressed traumatic memories that seemed
to lie at the root of the pathology had to do with sexual experiences.
Freud's attention became increasingly focused on the importance of
these early sexual experiences, usually recalled in the form of a sexual seduction occurring before puberty and often rather early in the
child's experience. Freud began to feel that these seduction experiences
were of central importance for the understanding of the etiology of
psychoneurosis. Over a period of several years, he continued to collect
clinical material that seemed to reinforce this important hypothesis.
He even went so far as to distinguish between the nature of the seductive experiences that were involved in hysterical manifestations and
those that were involved in obsessional neurosis. In the case of hysteria, he felt, the seduction experience had been primarily passive; that
is, the child had been the passive object of seductive activity on the
part of an adult or older child. In obsessive-compulsive neurosis, however, he felt the seduction experience had been an active one on the
part of the child. Thus, the child would have actively and aggressively
pursued a precocious sexual experience.

What was significant in all of this development was that Freud
had taken literally the accounts his patients had given him in the
form of forgotten but revived memories of such sexual involvement.
The patients provided him with "tales of outrage" that had been
committed by such relatives or caretakers as fathers, nursemaids, or
uncles. Freud had devoted little attention to the role of the child's
own psychological experience in the elaboration of these tales. Little
by little, Freud began to have some second thoughts about these so-
called memories. Several factors contributed to his doubt. First, he
had gained additional insight into the nature of pathological processes as a result of his clinical experience and his increasing awareness
of the role of fantasy in childhood. Second, he simply found it hard
to believe that there could be so many wicked and seductive adults
in Viennese society. The third influence, however, which undoubtedly
was of major significance in this reconsideration, was his own self-
analysis.

Freud had become increasingly aware of the importance of inner
processes. While he was attempting to come to terms with the subjective experience of his own patients, he also found himself drawn

to look inward and to find within his own introspective experience the reflections of what he had been able to identify in his patients. He began, therefore, the laborious process of his own self-analysis. He was able to survey his own history, to revive repressed memories from quite early levels of his childhood experience, and to begin to focus particular attention on the content of dreams; that is, both the dreams provided by his patients and those of his own experience.

As this important process of self-analysis progressed, Freud began to have more and more reason to call the seduction hypothesis into question. During this time, from 1893 to 1897, Freud was still using the combined technique of pressure and suggestion with relatively great assurance. Often he would insist that patients recall the seduction scene, so that much of the evidence on which the seduction hypothesis was based was open to the charge of suggestion. Consequently, as Freud became more aware of the role of suggestion in his technique, his doubts about the seduction hypothesis grew apace. In September 1897, his doubts came to a focus, and he wrote to his good friend Wilhelm Fliess as follows:

> Let me tell you straight away the great secret which has been slowly dawning on me in recent months. I no longer believe in my *neurotica*. That is hardly intelligible without an explanation; you yourself found what I told you credible. So I shall start at the beginning and tell you the whole story of how the reasons for rejecting it arose. The first group of factors were the continual disappointment of my attempts to bring my analyses to a real conclusion, the running away of people who for a time had seemed my most favourably inclined patients, the lack of the complete success on which I had counted, and the possibility of explaining my partial successes in other, familiar, ways. Then there was the astonishing thing that in every case . . . blame was laid on perverse acts by the father, and realization of the unexpected frequency of hysteria, in every case of which the same thing applied, though it was hardly credible that perverted acts against children were so general. . . . Thirdly, there was the definite realization that there is no "indication of reality" in the unconscious, so that it is impossible to distinguish between truth and emotionally charged fiction. (This leaves open the possible explanation that sexual fantasy regularly

makes use of the theme of the parents.) Fourthly, there was the consideration that even in the most deep-reaching psychoses the unconscious memory does not break through, so that the secret of infantile experiences is not revealed even in the most confused states of delirium. When one thus sees that the unconscious never overcomes the resistance of the conscious, one must abandon the expectation that in treatment the reverse process will take place to the extent that the conscious will fully dominate the unconscious. [*Origins*, pp. 215–216]

It is obvious that at this period Freud was struggling with his own great reluctance to abandon the seduction hypothesis. The doubts and the clarifying realization that he expressed to Fliess were depressing. After all, he had put in years of effort and had compiled a significant amount of evidence to bolster this seduction hypothesis. It was only with reluctance that he could surrender it. He also sensed, however, that in surrendering the seduction hypothesis, new possibilities for psychological exploration were opened up. In fact this juncture in the development of Freud's thinking was crucial. The abandonment of the seduction hypothesis, with its reliance on actual physical seduction, forced Freud to turn with new realization to the inner fantasy life of the child.

It can be said, in the real sense, that this shift from an emphasis on reality factors to an attention to and an understanding of the influence of inner motivations and fantasy products marks the real beginning of the psychoanalytic movement. In this attempt to distinguish psychic reality and fantasy from actual external events, and psychoneurosis from perversion, psychoanalysis itself took on a new and highly significant dimension. What inevitably emerged from this shift in direction was a dynamic theory of infantile sexuality in which the child's own psychosexual life played the significant and dominant role. This notion would replace the more static point of view in which the child represented an innocent victim whose eroticism was prematurely disrupted at the hands of unscrupulous adults.

The turning point was one of extreme significance for Freud himself. Increasingly, he turned his attention to his own self-analysis and put increasing reliance on it. He wrote to Fliess: "My self-analysis is the most important thing I have in hand, and promises to be of the greatest value to me, when it is finished" (*Origins*, p. 221).

More and more, he became involved in the study of dreams, all the more so as he developed the technique of free association, which provided him with a tool for exploring the associative content that underlies the dream experience. He concerned himself ever more so with the nature of infantile sexuality and with the inner sources of fantasy and dream content, namely, the unconscious instinctual drives. The abandonment of the seduction hypothesis was thus a crucial point in Freud's own development and the development of psychoanalysis, for it brought to an end the period of initial exploration and opened up the way to the development of psychoanalysis as it is known today.

Summary of the Beginnings—1887–1897

By 1897, when the hypothesis of actual seduction had fallen in the dust at Freud's feet, there had been a number of significant accomplishments. The fundamental concepts of psychic determinism and the operation of a dynamic unconscious were established, and concomitantly, a theory of psychoneurosis based on the idea of psychic conflict and the repression of disturbing childhood experiences had become clearly established. Sexuality, particularly in the form of childhood sexuality, had been unveiled as playing a significant but previously underplayed or ignored role in the production of psychological symptoms. More significantly, perhaps, Freud had arrived at a technique, a method of investigation, that could be exploited as a means of exploring a wide range of mental phenomena that had been poorly understood before Freud's time. Moreover, the horizons of psychoanalytic interest had begun to expand rapidly. Freud's attention was no longer focused on certain limited forms of psychopathology. It had begun to reach out, reflecting the wide-ranging curiosity and interests of Freud's mind, to embrace the understanding of dreams, creativity, wit and humor, the psychopathology of everyday experience, and a host of other normal and culturally significant mental phenomena. Psychoanalysis had indeed come to life.

THREE

Interpretation of Dreams

CURRENTLY, THE whole area of dream activity is one of the most exciting and intensely studied aspects of psychological functioning. The discovery of rapid-eye-movement (REM) cycles and the definition of the various stages of the sleep cycle have stimulated an intense and extremely productive flurry of research activity. A whole new realm of fresh and important questions has been opened up as a result of this activity, and psychoanalysts are drawing much closer to a more comprehensive understanding of the links between patterns of dream activity and underlying physiological and psychodynamic variables. As more is learned about this fascinating and complex problem, one comes much closer to understanding the nature of the dream process and to understanding the dream experience itself.

In this context it is difficult to look back and to appreciate the uniqueness and originality of Freud's immersion in the dream experience. It was only when Freud's attention had been refocused to the significance of inner fantasy experiences, by reason of the abandonment of the seduction hypothesis and in the context of his development of the technique of free association, that the significance and value of the investigation of dreams impressed itself on him. Freud became aware of the significance of dreams in his experience with his patients when he realized that, in the process of free association, his patients would frequently report their dreams along with the associative material that seemed connected with them. He discovered little by little that dreams had a definite meaning, although that meaning was often quite hidden and disguised. Moreover, when he encouraged his patients to associate freely to the dream fragments, Freud found that what they reported frequently was more productive of pertinent, repressed material than the associations to the events of their waking experience. Somehow the dream content seemed to be closer to the unconscious memories and fantasies of the repressed material, and the association to dream material seemed to facilitate the disclosure of this content.

Of central importance in this development of his thinking, and in the focusing on dream processes as an area of investigation, was Freud's self-analysis. Increasingly in the work of self-analysis, Freud relied on an examination and an associative exploration of his own dream experiences. More and more, through the years since the publication of *The Interpretation of Dreams,* the appreciation of the significance of Freud's self-analytic work has grown. It has become evident that many of the significant and revealing dreams presented in the dream book were actually Freud's own, although frequently not reported as such, and were the product of his self-analysis. This fact makes the monumental achievement of *The Interpretation of Dreams* all the more astounding.

Theory of Dreaming

The rich complex of data derived from Freud's clinical exploration of his patients' dreams and the profound insights derived from his associated investigation of his own dreams were distilled into the landmark publication in 1900 of *The Interpretation of Dreams.* Basing his analysis on these data, Freud presented a theory of the dream that paralleled his analysis of psychoneurotic symptoms. The dream was viewed as a conscious expression of an unconscious fantasy or wish not readily accessible to conscious waking experience. Thus, dream activity was considered as one of the normal manifestations of unconscious processes.

Freud felt that the dreaming experience of any normal person bore a significant resemblance to the pathological conscious organization of the thought processes in psychotic patients. The dream images

represented the unconscious wishes or thoughts, disguised through a
process of symbolization and other distorting mechanisms. This reworking of unconscious contents constituted the dream work. Freud
postulated the existence of a "censor," pictured as guarding the border
between the unconscious part of the mind and the preconscious
level. The censor functioned to exclude unconscious wishes during
conscious states but, during the regressive relaxation of sleep, allowed
certain unconscious contents to pass the border, yet only after transformation of the unconscious wishes into the disguised form experienced in the dream contents by the sleeping subject. Freud assumed
that the censor worked in the service of the ego; that is, he considered
it as serving the self-preservative objectives of the ego. Although the
mechanisms of the dream work, specifically the processes of displacement, condensation, symbolism, and repression, were originally identified in connection with the censor, Freud later attributed them to
the ego and superego of the structural theory, that is, as aspects of the
waking functioning of these parts of the mind and not specific to the
state of sleep and dreaming. While Freud was aware of the unconscious nature of the processes, he tended to regard the ego at this point
in the development of his theory more restrictively as the source of conscious processes of reasonable control and volition. We should not forget that, even in the *Studies on Hysteria*, repression was still envisioned
in intentional and volitional terms. His deepened appreciation of the
unconscious dimension of these processes led him to view the ego as in
some part unconscious, resulting in his formulation of the structural
theory in 1923.

Analysis of Dream Content

Freud's view of the dream material was that it contained content
that has been repressed or excluded from consciousness by the defensive activities of the ego. These activities during sleep were part
of the functions of the censor. The dream material, as it is consciously
recalled by the dreamer, is simply the end result of the unconscious
mental activity that takes place during sleep. Freud felt that the upsurge of unconscious material was so intense that it would threaten to
interrupt sleep itself, so that he envisioned the function of the censor
to be in part that of a guardian of sleep. Instead of being awakened by

these ideas, the sleeper dreams. Freud regarded the conscious experience of such thoughts during sleep as dreaming.

From a more contemporary viewpoint, it is known that the cognitive activity during sleep has a great deal of variety in it. Some of the
cognitive activity follows the description that Freud has provided of
dream activity, but much of it is considerably more realistic and more
consistently organized along logical lines. The dreaming activity that
Freud analyzed and described is probably more or less associated with
the stage 1 REM periods of the sleep-dream cycle.

The so-called manifest dream that embodies the experienced content of the dream, which the sleeper may or may not be able to recall
after waking, is the product of the dream activity. The unconscious
thoughts and wishes that in Freud's view threaten to awaken the
sleeper are described as the "latent dream content." Freud referred to
the unconscious mental operations by which the latent dream content
was transformed into the manifest dream as the "dream work." In the
process of dream interpretation, Freud was able to move from the
manifest content of the dream by way of associative exploration to
arrive at the latent dream content that lay behind the manifest dream
and that provided it with its core meaning.

In Freud's view there were a variety of stimuli that initiated dreaming activity. The contemporary understanding of the dream process,
however, would suggest that dreaming activity takes place more or
less in conjunction with the psychic patterns of central nervous acti-
vation that characterize certain phases of the sleep cycle. What Freud
thought to be initiating stimuli may in fact not be initiating at all but
may be merely incorporated into the dream content—and determine
to that extent the material in the dream thoughts.

Nocturnal Sensory Stimuli

A variety of such sensory impressions as pain, hunger, thirst, or
urinary urgency may play a role in determining dream content. Thus,
instead of disturbing one's sleep and leaving a warm bed, a sleeper
who is in a cold room and who urgently needs to urinate may dream of
awaking, voiding, and returning to bed. Freud's view would have been
that the activity of dreaming preserved and safeguarded the continuity of sleep. It is known now, however, that the function of dreaming is considerably more complex and cannot be regarded simply as

preserving sleep, although there is still room for this process to be counted among the dream functions.

Day Residues

Freud felt that one of the important elements that contributed to the shaping of the dream thoughts was the residue of thoughts and ideas and feelings that were left over from the experiences of the preceding day. These residues remain active in the unconscious and, like sensory stimuli, can be incorporated by the sleeper into the thought content of the manifest dream. Thus, the day residue could be amalgamated with the unconscious infantile drives and wishes that derive from the level of unconscious instincts. The amalgamation of infantile drives with elements of the day's residues effectively disguise the infantile impulse and allow it to remain effective as the driving force behind the dream. Day residues may in themselves be quite superficial or trivial, but they acquire their significance as dream instigators through the unconscious connections with deeply repressed instinctual drives and wishes.

Repressed Infantile Drives

Although these various elements may be determining aspects of the thought content of the dream experience, the essential elements of the latent dream content derive from one or several impulses emanating from the repressed part of the unconscious. In Freud's schema, the ultimate driving forces behind the dream activity and the process of dream formation were the wishes, originating in drives, stemming from an infantile level of psychic development. These drives take their content specifically from the oedipal and preoedipal levels of psychic integration. Thus, nocturnal sensation and the day residue play only an indirect role in determining dream content. A nocturnal stimulus, however intense, must be associated with and connected with one or more repressed wishes from the unconscious to give rise to the dream content. Moreover, Freud felt that unless a strong link between the day residue and the repressed content was established, the concerns of waking life would be unable of themselves to provide the impetus to dreaming activity no matter how compelling the claim on the sleeper's interests and attention in the waking state. This point of view needs some revision because it seems that in some phases of nighttime cognitive activity the mind is able to process the residues of daytime experience without much indication of connection with unconscious repressed content. However, in the phases of cognitive activity during sleep that bear the stamp of the dreaming activity as Freud has described and defined it, this essential link to the repressed probably still retains its validity.

Significance of Dreams

Once Freud's attention had definitively shifted to the study of inner processes of fantasy and dream formation, the study of dreams and the process of their formation became the primary route by which he gained access to the understanding of unconscious processes and their operation. Consequently, even to this day, Freud's monumental work *The Interpretation of Dreams* remains the standard source for the documentation and explanation of these unconscious processes that specifically come under the heading of primary process. In *The Interpretation of Dreams* he maintained that every dream somehow represents a wish fulfillment. He bolstered this hypothesis with a considerable amount of documentation, including exhaustive analysis of his own dreams.

There is a more general tendency today to view the dream activity as expressing a broader spectrum of psychological processes, keeping the aspect of wish fulfillment as one of the primary dimensions of dream activity, but not feeling it necessary to maintain it as an absolute principle, as it seemed to be in Freud's thinking. The manifest dream content seems to represent most clearly the imaginary fulfillment of a wish or impulse in early childhood, before such wishes have undergone repression. In later childhood, and even later in adulthood, however, the ego acts to defend itself against the unacceptable instinctual demands of the unconscious. These demands remain repressed to a large extent during the waking state, but in the regressive relaxation of the sleep state, the activity of the censor is somewhat more relaxed, so that the repressed impulses are allowed a greater degree of expression and become incorporated in a disguised and mutilated fashion in the manifest dream content. Nevertheless, the dream remains essentially a form of gratification of an unconscious instinctual impulse in fantasy form. In the state of suspended motility and regressive relaxation induced by sleep, the dream permits a partial and less dangerous gratification of the instinctual impulse.

This crucial aspect of wish fulfillment in the dream process is usually quite obscured by the extensive distortions and disguises brought about by the dream work, so that it often cannot be readily identified on a superficial examination of the manifest content. Inevitably, just as Freud's theory of neurosis has found an unsympathetic reception from those workers who have not accepted his findings concerning infantile sexuality, his theory of dreams has been rejected by those critics who tend to limit the focus of their investigations to the manifest elements of the dream content.

The Dream Work

The theory of the nature of the dream work, which Freud developed in *The Interpretation of Dreams,* became the fundamental description of the operation of unconscious processes—the basic mechanisms and the manner of their operating—that stands even today as an unsurpassed and foundational account of unconscious mental functioning. The focus of Freud's analysis was on the process by which the unconscious latent dream thoughts were disguised and distorted in such a fashion as to permit their expression and translation into the conscious manifest content of the dream. However, these unconscious processes, which were part of the fruit of his investigation, found ready application and extrapolation not only to the understanding of the formation of neurotic symptoms but, more broadly, to a whole range of unconscious productivity. The theory of dream work consequently became the basis for a wide-ranging analysis of unconscious operations that found expression in Freud's study of everyday experiences, as well as artistic creativity, jokes and humor, and a variety of culturally based activities of the human mind.

Representability

The basic problem of dream formation is to determine how it is that the latent dream content can find a means of representation in the manifest content. As Freud saw it, the state of sleep brought with it a relaxation of repression, and concomitantly, the latent unconscious wishes and impulses were permitted to press for discharge and gratification. Because the pathway to motor expression was blocked in the sleep state, these repressed wishes and impulses had to find other means of representation by way of the mechanisms of thought and fantasy. This representation was achieved in one of two ways. First of all, the thoughts, impressions, or memories that were suitable for representing these latent wishes and impulses in visual terms had to be provided. Individual experience in the course of the waking period provided an ample supply of such material. When current psychological experience could be linked with the repressed urges, it was incorporated into the content of the dream thoughts in the form of day residues. Similarly, nocturnal stimuli could be associated with repressed impulses and wishes and consequently give rise in the manifest content to representations in the form of auditory, tactile, olfactory, or gustatory elements.

The unconscious instinctual impulses that continually pushed for discharge had been repressed because of their unacceptable or painful nature. The activity of the dream censor provided a continual resistance to the discharge of these impulses, with the result that the impulses had to be attached to more neutral or "innocent" images to be able to pass the scrutiny of censorship and be allowed into conscious expression. This displacement was made possible by selecting apparently trivial or insignificant images from the residues of the individual's current psychological experience and linking these trivial images dynamically with the latent unconscious images, presumably on the basis of some resemblance that allowed the associative links to be established. In the process of facilitating the economic expression of latent unconscious contents and, at the same time, of maintaining the distortion that was essential for the contents to escape the repressing action of the censor, the dream work used a variety of mechanisms, making it possible for more neutral images to represent the repressed infantile components. These mechanisms included symbolism, displacement, condensation, projection, and secondary revision (Figure 2).

Symbolism

Symbolism is a complex process of indirect representation that in the psychoanalytic usage has the following connotations: (1) A sym-

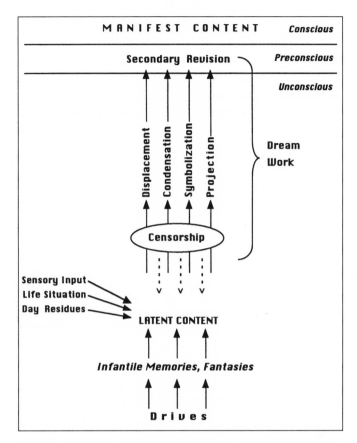

Figure 2.   Freud's (1990) view of the dream process [modified from Ellenberger]. In 1923 Freud altered his view of secondary revision, saying that, "strictly speaking," it was not part of the dream work.

bol is representative of or substitute for some other idea from which it derives a secondary significance that it does not possess of itself. (2) A symbol represents this primary element by reason of a common element that they share. (3) A symbol is characteristically sensory and concrete in nature, as opposed to the idea it represents, which may be relatively abstract and complex. A symbol thus provides a more condensed expression of the idea represented. (4) Symbolic modes of thought are more primitive, both ontogenetically and phylogenetically, and represent a form of regression to an earlier stage of mental development. Consequently, symbolic representations tend to function in more regressed conditions: in the thinking of primitive peoples, in myths, in states of poetic inspiration, and particularly in dreaming. (5) A symbol is thus a manifest expression of an idea that is more or less hidden or secret. Typically, the use of the symbol and its meaning is unconscious. Thus, symbols tend to be used spontaneously, automatically, and unconsciously. The use of symbols is a sort of secret language in which instinctually determined content can be reexpressed as other images; for example, money can symbolize feces, or windows can symbolize the female genitals.

In his examination of dream content, Freud discovered that the ideas or objects represented in this way were highly charged with inappropriate feelings and burdened with conflict. It was the forbidden meanings of these symbols, derived from instinctual impulses and urges, that remained unconscious. Freud toyed with the thought that symbols were somehow universal and inherited—following his notions of Lamarckian evolution—but he came gradually to attribute the use of such symbols to the basic similarities of interests and experiences in infancy. The common subjects dealt with in such forms of symbolic representations are usually body parts and functions, family members, birth, and death. Therefore, although the symbol disguises what is unacceptable, it can also offer partial gratification of underlying wishes or signify, and thus partially retain, lost objects.

Many questions still persist about the origins of symbolic processes, the stage of development in which they become organized, the extent to which they require altered states of consciousness such as the sleep state for their implementation, and the degree to which symbolic expression is related to underlying conflicts. Current formulations would regard the symbolic function as a uniquely human trait that is involved in all forms of human mental activity, from the most primitive expression of infantile wishes to the most complex creative processes of literary and artistic as well as scientific thinking.

Displacement

The mechanism of displacement refers to the transfer of amounts of energy (cathexis) from an original object to a substitute or symbolic representation of the object. Because the substitute object is relatively neutral—that is, less invested with affective energy—it is more acceptable to the dream censor and can pass the borders of repression more easily. Thus, whereas symbolism can be taken to refer to the substitution of one object for another, displacement facilitates the distortion of unconscious wishes through the transfer of affective energy from one object to another. Despite the transfer of cathectic energy, the aim of the unconscious impulse remains unchanged. For example, in a dream, the mother may be represented visually by an unknown female figure (at least one who has less emotional significance for the dreamer), but the naked content of the dream nonetheless continues to derive from the dreamer's unconscious instinctual impulses toward the mother. The role of displacement in the dream work is not to be underestimated; perhaps the greatest part of the distortion of dream content, which permits the latent impulses and wishes to be translated into manifest dream content, is accomplished by way of the mechanism of displacement.

Condensation

Condensation is the mechanism by which several unconscious wishes, impulses, or attitudes can be combined and attached to a single image in the manifest dream content. Thus, in a child's nightmare, an attacking monster may come to represent not only the dreamer's father, but may also represent some aspects of the mother and even, in addition, some of the child's own primitive hostile impulses as well. The converse of condensation can also occur in the dream work, namely, an irradiation or diffusion of a single latent wish or impulse that is distributed through multiple representations in the manifest dream content. The combination of mechanisms of condensation and diffusion provides the dreamer with a highly flexible and economic device for facilitating, compressing, and diffusing or expanding the manifest dream content, which is derived from the latent or unconscious wishes and impulses.

Projection

The process of projection allows dreamers to perceive their own unacceptable wishes or impulses as emanating in the dream from other persons or independent sources. Not surprisingly, the figures to whom

these unacceptable impulses are ascribed in the dream often turn out
to be the figures toward whom the subject's own unconscious impulses
are directed. For example, the individual who has a strong repressed
wish to be unfaithful to his wife may dream that his wife has been
unfaithful to him; or a patient may dream that she has been sexually
approached by her analyst, although she is reluctant to acknowledge
her own repressed wishes toward the analyst. Similarly, the child who
dreams of a destructive monster may be unable to acknowledge his
or her own destructive impulses and the fear of the father's power to
hurt the child. The figure of the monster consequently would be a
result of both projection and displacement.

Secondary Revision

The mechanisms of symbolism, displacement, condensation, and
projection are all characteristic of relatively early modes of cognitive
organization in a developmental sense. They reflect and express the
operation of the primary process, as will be shown. In the organization of the manifest dream content, however, the operation of primary process forms of organization is supplemented by a final process
that organizes the absurd, illogical, and bizarre aspects of the dream
thoughts into a more logical and coherent form. The distorting effects
of symbolism, displacement, and condensation thus acquire a coherence and rationality that is necessary for acceptance on the part of
the subject's more mature and reasonable ego through a process of secondary revision. Secondary revision thus uses intellectual processes
that more closely resemble organized thought processes governing
states of consciousness. It is through the process of secondary revision,
then, that the logical mental operations characteristic of the secondary
process are introduced into and modify dream work.

Affects in the Dream Work

In the process of displacement, condensation, symbolization, or
projection, the energic component of the instinctual impulses is separated from its representational component and undergoes an independent variety of vicissitudes. These drive aspects are expressed in the
form of affects or emotions.

The repressed emotion may not appear in the manifest dream content at all, or it may be experienced in a considerably altered form. Thus, for example, repressed hostility or hatred toward another individual may be modified into a feeling of annoyance or mild irritation in the manifest dream expression, or it may even be represented by an awareness of not being annoyed; that is, a conversion of the affect into its absence. The latent affect may possibly be directly transformed into an opposite in the manifest content, for example, as when a repressed longing might be represented by a manifest repugnance or vice versa. Thus, the vicissitudes of affect and the transformation by which latent affects are disguised introduce another dimension of distortion into the content of the manifest dream. The vicissitudes of affect, then, take place in addition to and in parallel with the processes of indirect representation that characterized the vicissitudes of dream content.

When Freud came to formulate his basic theory of dreams, he had by no means developed a comprehensive theory of the ego and its development and functions. Consequently, in his early studies of the dream process, he emphasized the role of the dream in discharging or gratifying instinctual wishes or impulses by the representation of wish fulfillments in the hallucinatory content of the dream. The same processes, however, can be looked at in light of their function of avoiding tension or psychic pain. This is essentially a defensive function and is properly the domain of the ego. The dream thus affords an opportunity for studying some of the important if more primitive functions of the ego. It was only gradually that Freud realized that processes of symbol formation, displacement, condensation, projection, and secondary revision all serve a dual purpose. If they facilitate the discharge of unconscious drive impulses, they also may be regarded as primitive defense mechanisms that prevent the direct discharge of instinctual drives. They thereby protect the dreamer from an excessive discharge of unconscious impulses and from the excessive anxiety and pain that would accompany it.

These mechanisms, however, have only a limited capacity to disguise and channel unconscious instinctual drive derivatives. When anxiety pervades the dream content or becomes so severe that it forces at least a partial awakening, this suggests some failure in the primitive defensive operations of the ego. An element of the latent dream content has succeeded, despite the dream work and the repressing efforts of the censor, in forcing its way into the manifest dream content in a form that is too direct, too little disguised, and too readily recognized for the ego to tolerate it. The ego reacts to this direct expression of repressed impulses with anxiety. Incidentally, even in *The Interpretation of Dreams* Freud foreshadowed a later development in his thinking about anxiety; namely, that the censor seemed to serve a warning function that alerted the ego to the breakthrough of instinctual and repressed impulses. This warning function was formalized later in Freud's theory of signal anxiety.

The punishment dream is related to the anxiety dream. In the punishment dream, the ego anticipates a condemnation on the part of the superego (conscience) if a part of the latent content, which derived from repressed impulses, should find its direct expression in the manifest dream content. Specifically, in reaction to the anticipation of the dire consequences of the loss of ego control in sleep and the threat of instinctual breakthrough, there is developed a compromise between the repressed wish and the repressing agency, specifically the superego. Thus, the demands of the superego for punishment are satisfied in the dream content by giving expression to punishment fantasies. It is to be noted that, in dealing with these various vicissitudes of dream functioning, Freud was formulating in a preliminary and as yet unselfconscious way some of the parameters of the mental apparatus that would find more explicit and sophisticated expression in his tripartite (structural) theory.

FOUR

Psychic Apparatus and Topographic Theory

IN HIS FAMOUS seventh chapter in *The Interpretation of Dreams*, Freud surveyed the copious information he had gathered about dreaming processes and specifically focused his ideas on the nature of dream work. In addition, he provided a model of the psychic apparatus as he understood it at the turn of the century. Not only was the model he proposed a description of the functioning of the dreaming mind, but it also represented a broader conceptualization of the psychic apparatus as it functioned through the range of both pathological and normal human experience. What is most striking about this model from a present-day perspective is that it represents an elaborate attempt to recast in more psychological language the basic model of the mind that Freud had formulated first in his *Project for a Scientific Psychology*. It seems clear that the economic model, which Freud expended such intense effort on in the 1890s and seemingly had abandoned in frustration, had come back to reassert itself, now in a new language and in a different setting. The lines of continuity and the parallels between the model of the *Project* and the model of the seventh chapter could not be appreciated until the manuscript of the *Project* was rediscovered after Freud's death.

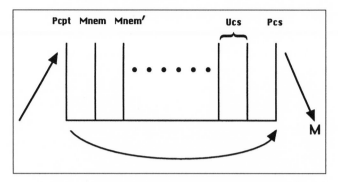

Figure 3.　Freud's 1900 model of the psychic apparatus

Psychic Apparatus—1900

The model that Freud presented in 1900 was, taken schematically, an elaborate construction based on a basic notion of a stimulus-response mechanism (Figure 3). In normal waking experience the sensory input was taken into the receptor end of the apparatus and was then processed in a number of mnemonic systems of increasing degrees of elaborateness and complexity. After varying degrees of processing, the impulse was subsequently discharged through the motor effector apparatus. In the dream state the motor effector pathways were blocked so that, instead of discharge through motor effector systems, the excitation was forced to move in a backward or regressive direction through the mnemonic systems and back into the sensory systems.

During the daytime the path leading from the unconscious levels of the apparatus through the preconscious to conscious levels was barred to the dream thoughts by the activity of the censor. In sleep, however, this pathway was again available because the resistance of the censor was diminished in sleep. Consequently, unconscious memories and their instinctual determinants could press to discharge through the perceptual apparatus, as was particularly the case in hallucinatory dream experiences. Thus, dreams could be described as having a regressive character. Consisting specifically in the turning back of an idea into the sensory image from which it was originally derived, regression was an effect of resistance opposing the discharge of energy associated with the thought into consciousness along the normal path. Regression was also contributed to by simultaneous attraction exercised on the thought by the presence of associated memories in the unconscious.

In the case of dreams, regression is further facilitated by the diminution of the progressive current that flows from the continuing sensory input during waking hours. Regression, as Freud viewed it, was essentially a regression to the originating source of an impression as he described it in the reversal within the mental apparatus, but it also was a regression in time. He commented:

> Nor can we leave the subject of regression in dreams without setting down in words a notion by which we have already repeatedly been struck and which will recur with fresh intensity when we have entered more deeply into the study of the psychoneurosis: namely that dreaming is on the whole an example of regression to the dreamer's earliest condition, a revival of his childhood, of the instinctual impulses which dominated it and of the methods of expression which were then available to him. [5 *SE* 548]

Freud distinguished several forms of regression; namely, a *topographic regression* that involved a regression in the ψ-systems within the mental model; a *temporal regression* according to which the mental process refers back to older psychical structures, particularly those deriving from an infantile level of development; and *formal regression*, in which more primitive methods of expression and representation take the place of the more normal ones. "All these three kinds of regression," Freud commented, "are, however, one at bottom and occur together as a rule; for what is older in time is more primitive in form and in psychical topography lies nearer to the perceptual end" (5 *SE* 548).

Perhaps the most central aspect of the functioning of this mental model, and the aspect of it that comes strikingly close to the formulations of the *Project*, has to do with Freud's notions of the primary and secondary processes. To begin with, the impulses and instinctual wishes originating in infancy served as the indispensable nodal force for dream formation. The energic conception of these drives followed the basic economic principles laid down by the *Project* (Table 1). They were elevated states of psychic tension in which the energy was constantly seeking discharge according to the constancy principle and the pleasure principle, which Freud had previously formulated.

The tendency to discharge, however, was opposed by other psychic systems. Thus, Freud envisioned two fundamentally different kinds of psychic processes involved in the formation of dreams. One of these processes tended to produce a rational organization of dream thoughts, which was of no less validity in terms of contact with reality than normal thinking. However, another system—the first psychic system in Freud's schema—treated the dream thoughts in a bewildering and irrational manner. He felt that a more normal train of thought could only be submitted to abnormal psychic treatment if an unconscious wish, derived from infancy and in a state of repression, had been transferred onto it. As a result of the operation of the pleasure principle, the first psychic system was incapable of bringing anything disagreeable into the context of the dream thoughts. It was unable to do anything but wish. Operating in conjunction with the demands of this primary system, the secondary system could only cathect an unconscious idea if it could inhibit any development of unpleasure that might have proceeded from the bringing to awareness of that idea. Anything that might evade that inhibition would be equivalently inaccessible to the second system, as well as to the first, because it would promptly be eliminated in accordance with the unpleasure principle.

The psychic process derived from the operation of the first system is referred to as "primary process," and it mirrors the primary process as described in the development of the *Project*. The process resulting from the inhibition imposed by the second system is referred to as the "secondary process," and it reflects the operation of the system of inhibition and delay sketched in the *Project*. The secondary system thus corrects and regulates the primary system. Among the wishful impulses derived from infantile impulses, there are some whose fulfillment would be a contradiction of the purposes and ideas of secondary process thinking. The fulfillment of these wishes could no longer generate an affect of pleasure, but would be unpleasurable. This formulation, it should be noted, formed the basis for Freud's later elaboration of the pleasure principle as opposed to the reality principle.

Thus, one can note the significant role that the mental model of *The Interpretation of Dreams* served in the development of Freud's thinking. It was, in a way, a résumé and recasting of the original economic model that Freud had developed in the *Project*. Similarly, in a forward-looking perspective, the model opens the way to the development of the instinct theory and the associated topographic model that dominated Freud's thinking for nearly the next quarter century.

Topographic Theory

Beginning with abandonment of the seduction hypothesis, with the concomitant turning of Freud's interests to the inner processes of fantasy and dream formation, and ending with the publication of *The Ego and the Id*, in 1923, in which Freud propounded his structural model of the psychic apparatus, Freud's thinking was dominated by the topographic theory. The shift from a seduction model, directing his curiosity and attention to the inner products of instinctual drives, unavoidably involved him in a concerted effort to understand and grasp in theoretical terms the nature of the underlying instinctual drives that were the motivating force behind these phenomena and that were related to and driving unconscious processes. The period from 1900 until 1923 saw a gradual evolution and development of Freud's ideas about instincts and a continuing reworking and enriching of his theory of instinctual drives.

Basic Assumptions

There were a number of assumptions underlying Freud's thinking and serving as lines of continuity between the various stages of his investigations. By means of these assumptions, the successive models around which his thinking organized itself were connected. The first assumption was that of "psychological determinism," which held that all psychological events, including behaviors, feelings, thoughts, and actions, are caused by—that is, are the end result of—a preceding sequence of causal events. This assumption was derived from Freud's Helmholtzian convictions and represents the application of a basic natural-science principle to psychological understanding; but it was also reinforced by Freud's clinical observation that apparently meaningless hysterical symptoms, which had been previously attributed to somatic etiology, could be relieved by relating them to past, apparently repressed, experiences. Thus, apparently arbitrary pathological

behavior could be tied into a causal psychological network. This observation was the empirical point of departure for Freud's exploration
into other aspects of psychic functioning. The connection of psychological events with explanatory "causes" does not specifically address
the nature of psychological causes. Freud did not have in mind the distinction between causes and motives or reasons. Although his frame of
reference was to an extent committed to nonpsychological events as
the "causes" of all scientifically describable events, he nonetheless appealed to motives and meanings as part of the determinative sequence
in explaining the origins of symptoms. The inherent determinism of
psychoanalysis is generally accepted as resting on such psychological
causes involving motive and meaning, usually on an unconscious level.

The second assumption is that of "unconscious psychological processes." This assumption was derived from a considerable amount of
evidence that had been gathered through the use of hypnosis, but it
was also consolidated by Freud's experience of the free associating of
his patients bringing past experiences to awareness. The unconscious
material, which survived and was able to influence present experience,
was found to be governed by specific rules, for example, the pleasure
principle and the mechanisms of primary process that differed radically from those of conscious behavior and thought processes. Thus,
the unconscious processes were brought within the realm of psychological understanding and explanation.

The third assumption is that "unconscious psychological conflicts"
among forces form the basic elements at the root of psychoneurotic difficulties. This assumption was related to Freud's experience
of the resistance and the drive to repression in his patients. The full
realization of this aspect of psychic functioning came only with the
awareness that the reports of patients represented not unconscious
memories of actual experiences but, rather, unconscious fantasies. The
assumption of unconscious forces accounted for the process that created those fantasies and brought them into consciousness during free
association. It also accounted for the agency that opposed the coming
to consciousness of such fantasies. This counterforce that clashed with
the sexual drives and diverted them into fantasies or symptoms was related to the function of censorship in the dream theory and, later, to
the operation of ego instincts that were set in opposition to the sexual
instincts.

The final assumption of the topographic theory was that there existed "psychological energies" that originated in instinctual drives. This assumption was derived from the observation that recall of traumatic experiences and their accompanying affect resulted in the disappearance of symptoms and anxiety. It was suggested, therefore, that a displaceable and transformable quantity of energy was involved in the psychological processes responsible for symptom formation. Freud originally assumed that this quantity was the affect, which became dammed up or strangulated when it was not appropriately expressed and, thus, was transformed into anxiety or conversion symptoms. After he had developed his notion of instinctual drives, this quantitative factor was conceived of as drive energy (cathexis). As noted previously (in chapter 1), the assumption of psychic energies served Freud as an important heuristic metaphor. The usefulness of the metaphor and its necessity as a basic assumption of analytic theory are currently in question.

Topographic Model

Freud's thinking about the mental apparatus at this time was based on the classification of mental operations and contents according to regions or systems in the mind. These systems were described neither in anatomical nor spatial terms but were specified, rather, according to their relationship to consciousness. Any mental event that occurred outside of conscious awareness and that could not be made conscious by the effort of focusing attention was said to belong to the deepest regions of the mind, the unconscious region or system. Mental events that could be brought to conscious awareness through an act of attention were said to be preconscious and, consequently, were not to be regarded as derived from the deepest levels of the mind, the unconscious. The mental events that occurred in conscious awareness were regarded as belonging to the perceptual-consciousness system and were conceived of as located on the surface of the mind. The topographic model has essentially fallen into disuse because of limited utility as a working model of psychoanalytic processes, largely because it has been surpassed and supplanted by the structural theory. The topographic viewpoint, however, is still useful for classifying mental events descriptively by quality and degree of awareness.

Consciousness

The conscious system was that region of the mind in which the perceptions coming from the outside world or from within the body or the mind were brought into awareness. Internal perceptions could include observations of thought processes or affective states of various kinds. Consciousness is by and large a subjective phenomenon, the content of which can only be communicated by language or behavior. It has also been regarded psychoanalytically as a sort of superordinate sense organ, which can be stimulated by perceptual data impinging on the central nervous system. It is assumed that the function of consciousness uses a form of neutralized psychic energy, namely, "attention cathexis."

The nature of consciousness was described in less detail in Freud's early theories, and certain aspects of consciousness are not yet completely understood by psychoanalysts. Freud regarded the conscious system as operating in close association with the preconscious. Through attention, the subject could become conscious of perceptual stimuli from the outside world. From within the organism, however, only elements in the preconscious were allowed to enter consciousness. The rest of the mind lay outside awareness in the unconscious. Before 1923, however, Freud also believed that consciousness controlled motor activity and regulated the qualitative distribution of psychic energy.

The Preconscious

The preconscious system consists of those mental events, processes, and contents that are for the most part capable of reaching or being brought into conscious awareness by the act of focusing attention. The quality of preconscious organizations may range from reality-oriented thought sequences, or problem-solving analysis with highly elaborated secondary process schemata, all the way to more primitive fantasies, daydreams, or dream-like images, which reflect a more primary process organization. The term was originally applied by Freud to the mental contents capable of becoming conscious easily and under quite frequent conditions. Preconscious content normally reaches consciousness by an increase in cathexis mediated by attention. Thus, it stands over and against unconscious processes in which the transformation to consciousness is accomplished only with great difficulty and by dint of the expenditure of considerable energy in overcoming the barrier of repression.

The preconscious region of the mind is not present at birth but develops in childhood in a manner that parallels the course of ego development, as described in the later structural theory. The preconscious is accessible to both consciousness and the unconscious proper. Elements of the unconscious can only gain access to consciousness by first becoming linked with words and thus reaching the preconscious. One of the functions of the preconscious is to maintain the repressive barrier or censorship of wishes and desires. The secondary process organization of preconscious thinking is aimed at avoiding unpleasure, at delaying instinctual discharge, and at binding mental energy in accordance with the demands of external reality and the subject's moral principles or values. Thus, the functioning of the secondary process is closely connected with the reality principle and is governed, for the most part, by the dictates of the reality principle.

The Unconscious

Unconscious mental events, namely, those that are not within conscious awareness, can be described from one of several viewpoints. One can think of the unconscious *descriptively*; that is, as referring to the sum total of all mental contents and processes at any given moment outside of the range of conscious awareness, including those aspects of the mind that Freud referred to as preconscious.

One can also think of the unconscious *dynamically;* that is, as referring to those mental contents and processes that are incapable of achieving consciousness because of the operation of a counterforce, the force of censorship or repression. This repressive force or "counter-cathexis" manifests itself in psychoanalytic treatment as a resistance to remembering. The unconscious mental contents in this dynamic sense consist of drive representations or wishes that are in some measure unacceptable, threatening, or abhorrent to the intellectual or ethical standpoint of the individual. The drives are nonetheless regarded as continually striving for discharge in behavior or thought processes. This results in intrapsychic conflict between the repressed forces of the mind and the repressing forces. When the repressive countercathexis weakens, the result may be the formation of neurotic symptoms.

The symptom is thus viewed as essentially a compromise between conflicting forces. These unconscious mental contents are also organized on the basis of infantile wishes or drives, rather than logically or realistically. They also strive for immediate discharge, regardless of the reality conditions. Consequently, the dynamic unconscious is thought to be regulated by the demands of primary process and the pleasure principle.

Finally, there is a *systematic* sense of the unconscious that refers to a region or system within the organization of the mental apparatus that embraces the dynamic unconscious and within which memory traces are organized by primitive modes of association, as dictated by the primary process. This systematic view of the unconscious is considered, in a specific topographic sense, as a component subsystem within the topographic model. Consequently, the systematic unconscious can be described in terms of the following characteristics:

1. Ordinarily, the elements of the systematic unconscious are inaccessible to consciousness and can only become conscious through access to the preconscious, which excludes them by means of censorship or repression. Repressed ideas, consequently, may only reach consciousness when the censor is overpowered (as in psychoneurotic symptom formation), or relaxes (as in dream states), or is fooled (in jokes).

2. The unconscious system is exclusively associated with primary process thinking. The primary process has as its principal aim the facilitation of wish fulfillment and instinctual discharge. Consequently, it is intimately associated with—and functions as—the pleasure principle. As such, it disregards logical connections, permits contradictions to coexist simultaneously, recognizes no negatives, has no conception of time, and represents wishes as fulfillments. The unconscious system can also be recognized to use those primitive mental operations that Freud identified in the operation of the dream process (Figure 2). Thus, displacement and condensation permit rapid discharge of mental energies attached to repressive affects and ideas through the preconscious and conscious systems. As defined in the earlier consideration of dreams, displacement is the mechanism by which mental energy (cathexis) that is attached to one idea can be shifted to another idea that may en-

counter less censorship. Condensation is the process by which energy attached to more than one unconscious idea may be discharged through a single thought or image embodying (symbolically) the characteristics of these several ideas. Condensation thus introduces a property of economy in unconscious operations. Moreover, the quality of motility, which is characteristic of primary process thinking and of unconscious energy, is also frequently linked to the capacity for creative thinking.

3. Memories in the unconscious have been divorced from their connection with verbal symbols. Freud discovered in the course of his clinical work that repression of a childhood memory could occur if the energy was withdrawn from it and, especially, if the verbal energy was removed. When the words were reapplied to the forgotten memory traits (as during psychoanalytic treatment), it became recathected and could thus reach consciousness once more.

4. The content of the unconscious is limited to wishes seeking fulfillment. These wishes provide the motive force for dreams and neurotic symptom formation. It has already been noted that this view may be oversimplified.

5. The unconscious is closely related to the instincts. At this level of theory development, the instincts were considered to consist of sexual and self-preservative (ego) drives. The unconscious was thought of as containing the mental representatives and derivatives of the sexual instincts particularly.

Dynamics of Mental Functioning

Freud conceived of the psychic apparatus, in the context of the topographic model, as a kind of reflex arc in which the various segments have a spatial relationship (Figure 3). The arc consisted of a perceptual or sensory end through which impressions were received; an intermediate region, consisting of a storehouse of unconscious memories; and a motor end, closely associated with the preconscious, through which instinctual discharge could occur. In early childhood, perceptions were modified and stored in the form of memories.

According to this theory, in ordinary waking life the mental energy associated with unconscious ideas seeks discharge through thought or motor activity, moving from the perceptual end to the motor end.

Under certain conditions, such as external frustration or sleep, the direction in which the energy travels along the arc is reversed, and it moves from the motor end to the perceptual end. It thereby reanimates earlier childhood impressions in their earlier perceptual forms and results in dreams during sleep or hallucinations in mental disorders. This reversal of the normal flow of energy in the psychic apparatus was the "topographic regression" discussed previously. Although Freud subsequently abandoned this model of the mind as a reflex arc, the central concept of regression was retained and applied later in a somewhat modified form in the theory of neurosis. The theory states that libidinal frustration results in a reversion to earlier modes of instinctual discharge or levels of fixation, which had been previously determined by childhood frustrations or excessive erotic stimulations. Freud called this kind of reversion to instinctual levels of fixation libidinal or instinctual regression.

Framework of Psychoanalytic Theory:
Repressed versus the Repressing

Throughout his long lifetime and in the course of the many twistings and turnings of the theoretical developments in his thinking, Freud's mind was dominated by a tendency to describe many of the aspects of mental functioning as contrasting phenomena. Freud thought in terms of contrasting polarities; some of the primary polarities were that of subject (ego) versus object (outer world), pleasure versus unpleasure, and activity versus passivity. Thus, his thinking about mental operations was dominated by a basic dualism. The fundamental dualism that dominated his thinking during the long maturation of psychoanalytic ideas—and that still constitutes a basic dimension of psychoanalytic thinking—was the dualism that existed between the forces and contents of the mind that were viewed as repressed and unconscious and those forces and mental agencies that were responsible for the repression. Although the persistence of such basic dualism in psychoanalytic thinking has clear advantages and undoubtedly helps one understand some fundamental aspects of the mind, one should not forget that such paradigms may prove to be restrictive. There is real question in the current state of psychoanalysis as to whether some of these assumed basic dimensions may not in fact be limiting the capacity of psychoanalytic theory to grow apace with the expanding horizons of both clinical experience and experimental exploration. The historical role and the present vitality of the basic psychoanalytic dualism, however, should not be undervalued; it provides a powerful tool for understanding and treating clinical pathology.

In a basic sense psychoanalytic theory may be conveniently divided into a theory of the repressed, on one hand, and a theory of the repressing agency, on the other. Both of these aspects of analytic theory underwent progressive delineation and evolution, and in each case the evolution was relatively independent. Early in his thinking about this duality, and particularly in his focus on the fundamental clinical fact of intrapsychic conflict, Freud envisioned the duality as the conflict of opposing instinctual forces. Thus, he opposed the repressed sexual instincts to the repressing countercathectic force of the ego instincts. It was only gradually that his point of view shifted so that, instead of thinking in terms of countervailing instinctual forces, he envisioned the repressing agency as a regulatory psychic apparatus.

In the early years, however, his attention was taken up quite intently by the excitement of discovery in understanding the instinctual processes and drives themselves. It was only incrementally as the horizons of his clinical concern and theoretical interest broadened that he began to focus increasingly on the regulatory apparatus. This discussion will follow in his footsteps, as it were, and first consider that part of psychoanalytic theory dealing with the development of the sexual and aggressive instincts, in particular their source, aim, impetus, and object. Subsequently, that part of the theory concerned with the formation and function of the repressing psychic apparatus, currently referred to as ego psychology, will be considered.

Consequently, in a presentation such as this, in which the interests of pedagogy are served by dividing aspects of the theory and discussing their development separately, one needs constantly to recall that one is dealing with aspects of an integrated psychic organism and that the various aspects of its functioning cannot adequately be understood without reference to other parts of the theory.

FIVE

The Theory
of Instincts

ALL HUMAN BEINGS have similar instincts. The actual discharge of these instinctual impulses is organized, directed, regulated, or even repressed by the functions of the individual ego, which mediates between the organism and the external world. Historically, the detailed exploration of the instincts in psychoanalysis preceded Freud's preoccupation with ego psychology. There is also a logical sequence, however, because one would not try to investigate an apparatus whose function it was to organize, direct, regulate, and repress without having a prior understanding of the precise nature of the phenomena subjected to such organization, direction, and regulation. To an increasing extent, the study of the ego as a product of the interaction of unconscious instinctual demands and environmental influences has become a dominant concern not only of psychoanalysts but also of social scientists in allied disciplines. One of the dangers in this trend is that the increasing emphasis on ego psychology and its connections with more general psychological interests has been accompanied by an increasing theoretical separation between noninstinctual ego apparatuses and the unconscious motivating forces of the instincts. Thus, there is the risk of de-emphasizing the study of the deeper instinctual forces of the mind and of eclipsing elemental psychological processes, which may not be to the ultimate advantage of psychoanalytic understanding. With this in mind, one can turn now to the psychoanalytic instinct theory.

Concepts of Instincts

One of the first problems that must be dealt with in considering the theory of instincts is what is meant by the term "instinct." The problem is made more complex by the variation in usage between a primarily biological use and Freud's primarily psychological use. The difficulties are also compounded by the complexities in Freud's own use of the term.

The term "instinct" was introduced primarily by students of animal behavior. It refers generally to a pattern of species-specific behavior that is based mainly on the potentialities determined by heredity and is therefore considered to be relatively independent of learning. The term was applied to a great variety of behavior patterns, including patterns described in such terms as a maternal instinct, a nesting instinct, or a migrational instinct. Such usage resisted successful physiological explanation and tended to introduce a strong teleological connotation, thus implying some sense of purposefulness, as in the use of a concept of an instinct of self-preservation. Freud adopted this usage unquestioningly, but its validity has been questioned even by strong proponents of instinctual theory among animal behaviorists.

The utility of a concept of instinct has been undermined from at least two directions. From the side of evolutionary change and the theory of genetics, evolutionary change is regarded as taking place primarily through mutation and natural selection. Mutations having a greater survival value are thus transmitted by the genetic code and result in the survival of those species members who bear the particular qualities resulting from mutation. The teleological import of instincts as serving the interests of species survival are consequently limited. The other inroad on instinctual theory derives from increasing awareness from experimental study and more extensive natural observation of the modification of instinctual patterns through experiential learning. The dichotomy of nature-nurture can no longer be simplistically or rigidly maintained. Thus, instinctually derived patterns of behavior are seen to be increasingly modifiable in the interests of adaptation. Ethologists consequently prefer to speak simply of species-typical behavior patterns that are based on innate equipment but that mature and develop or are elicited through a certain degree of environmental interaction.

Freud, of course, took as the basis of his thinking the older concept of instinct, but in adopting it for his purposes he transformed it. Actually, Freud's own formulation of the notion of instinct underwent some shifting so that he actually offered a variety of definitions. Perhaps the most cogent was: "an 'instinct' appears to us as a concept on the frontier between the mental and the somatic, as the psychical representative of the stimuli originating from within the organism and reaching the mind, as a measure of the demand made upon the mind for work in consequence of its connection with the body" (14 *SE* 121–122). It can be seen immediately that the basic ambiguity in the concept of instinct between the biological and the psychological aspects continued to influence Freud's thinking about instinctual drives and remains latent in subsequent psychoanalytic usage of the term.

Freud himself varied in the emphasis he placed on one or other aspect of it, and the subsequent discussion of the concept of instinct in psychoanalysis has varied similarly between an emphasis on the biological aspects and an emphasis on the psychological aspects. The concept of instinct, then, standing on the borderline between the somatic and the psychic, embraces both the aspect of physiologically derived, organismic drive components, on one hand, and an aspect of mental representation that is specifically psychic, on the other. Psychoanalytic theorists, even on the contemporary scene, vary in the degree to which they think of these dual components as either integrated or separated. The instinct, then, is a psychic representation of internal stimuli, and the stimuli represent physiological needs. The physiological needs, as for example hunger, which can be described in such physiological process terms as lowering of blood sugar or emptying of the stomach, cannot be confused with the psychic representation, whether that representation be conscious, preconscious, or unconscious. Freud's notion of instinct, however, embraces all of these in varying degrees and with varying emphasis.

Another unfortunate source of confusion was that the term used by Freud was the German word *Trieb*. The term has usually been translated into English, especially in the normative *Standard Edition*, as "instinct." One might ask why *Trieb* was not simply translated as "drive"?

The reluctance to do this was apparently based on the fact that the drive concept had been rather widely abused in behavioral sciences. There was presumably a wish on the part of psychoanalytic theorists to maintain some distance between their own basic concepts and the notions of drive that were used by behavioral theorists. Moreover, Freud assumed that the *Triebe* were based on innate givens; that is, preformed biological potentials present at birth. This aspect of the concept was reflected in the English term "instinct." Nevertheless, in an attempt to avoid the semantic pitfalls involved in the term "instinct," general usage currently prefers to use the term "instinctual drive" to express the Freudian notion of *Trieb*.

Concept of Libido

The ambiguity in the term instinctual drive is reflected also in the usage of the term "libido." Briefly, Freud regarded the sexual instinct as a psychophysiological process that had both mental and physiological manifestations. Essentially, he used the term "libido" to refer to "[t]he force by which the sexual instinct is represented in the mind" (17 *SE* 137). Thus, in its accepted sense, "libido" refers specifically to the mental manifestations of the sexual instinct.

Freud recognized early that the sexual instinct did not originate in a finished or final form, as represented by the stage of genital primacy. Rather, it underwent a complete process of development at each phase of which the libido had specific aims and objects that diverged in varying degrees from the simple aim of genital union. The libido theory thus came to include the investigation of all of these manifestations and the complicated paths that they followed in the course of psychosexual development.

Infant Sexuality

It had long been supposed that Freud's thought on infantile sexuality constituted an assault on the cherished ideas of 19th-century and Victorian thinking and that he was violently attacked for his views of the erotic life of young children. It seems, however, that his significant contribution, the 1905 *Three Essays on the Theory of Sexuality,* came not as an exceptional work but as part of a flood of literature dealing with sexual problems. Contemporary sexual mores, particularly in the libertine atmosphere of Vienna, were quite lax, and there was hardly any aspect of sexual life, including the grossest perversions, that was not openly known and discussed. It is difficult to draw a line between Freud's sources and the parallel developments that were taking place in the intellectual climate around him. There was little in his psychosexual theory that was not already extant in the literature and usage of his time. The notions of infantile sexuality and the early phases of sexual development were by no means new. The notion of bisexuality had been anticipated by several decades. Freud's notion of anal eroticism seems to have been somewhat more original, but even there, elements of it had been anticipated. Even the concept of narcissism had been described and argued about. Ellenberger commented in 1970 on this aspect of Freud's theory:

> Current accounts of Freud's life state that the publication of his sexual theories aroused anger because of their unheard-of novelty in a "Victorian" society. Documentary evidence shows that this does not correspond to fact. Freud's *Three Essays* appeared in the midst of a flood of contemporary literature on sexology and were favorably received. Freud's main originality was to synthesize ideas and concepts, the majority of which lay scattered or partially organized, and to apply them directly to psychotherapy. [1970:508]

Nonetheless, it would not be unexpected that Freud's clear and rather forceful presentation of these ideas about the development of sexuality should not meet with some resistance. Some people have always found the undermining of the myth of childhood innocence to be difficult to accept. Even relatively sophisticated psychiatric residents today will at times react with incredulity to the elucidation of sexual material in clinical cases of childhood neuroses. As is so often the case in figures of great genius, however, Freud's contribution was not so much in originating the ideas about psychosexual development as in his capacity to integrate them in a consistent and coherent theory that brought them to bear on the understanding of clinical phenomena with which he was dealing in his patients.

Freud had become convinced of the relationship between sexual trauma, in both childhood traumata and the genesis of psychoneurosis, and disturbances of sexual functioning as related to the so-called actual neuroses; that is, hypochondriasis, neurasthenia, and anxiety neuroses. Freud originally viewed these conditions as related to misuse of sexual function. Thus, for example, anxiety neurosis was thought to be due to the inadequate discharge of sexual products, leading to the damming up of libido that was then converted into anxiety. Also, he attributed neurasthenia to excessive masturbation and a diminution in available libidinal energy. The actual neuroses will be discussed later on in the consideration of the development of Freud's ideas about anxiety. In any case, these studies had led Freud to an awareness of the importance of sexual factors in the etiology of psychoneurotic states.

As his clinical experience increased, Freud was able to reconstruct the early sexual experiences and fantasies of his patients. These data provided the framework for a developmental theory of childhood sexuality, which in the subsequent course of psychoanalytic exploration has been amply corroborated in many respects by direct observation of childhood behavior. In addition to the data he derived from his clinical experience, perhaps an even more important source of information that contributed to Freud's thinking about infantile sexuality was his own self-analysis that he had begun in 1897. He was gradually able to recover memories of his own erotic longings in childhood and his conflicts in relationship to his parents, related specifically to his oedipal involvement. The realization of the operation of such infantile sexual longings in his own experience suggested to Freud that these phenomena might not be restricted only to the pathological development of the neurosis, but that essentially normal individuals might undergo similar developmental experiences.

Freud had virtually completed his basic theoretical notions about the essential phases of sexual development before the turn of the century, but the publication of his synthesis of views on psychosexual development was delayed until 1905. It was then that *Three Essays on the Theory of Sexuality* saw the light of day in the first of many editions. It is somewhat surprising that the detailed discussion of sexual development of children, including the notions of pregenital organization of the libido, as well as the libido theory itself, first appeared in 1915 in the third edition of the *Three Essays*. Although Freud used the term "sexuality" in these essays in a more or less familiar sense to refer to the erotic life of the individual, he also extended the general concept to include those sensations and activities that could be described as sensual, in the sense that they were a source of pleasure and gratification, but were not generally considered as sexual. Freud was able to indicate through levels of development the connection between such sensual behaviors and activities and libidinal gratification.

Phases of Psychosexual Development

The earliest manifestations of infantile sexuality, as Freud described them in the *Three Essays*, arise in relation to bodily functions that are basically nonsexual, such as feeding and the development of bowel and bladder control. Therefore, Freud divided these stages of psychosexual development into a succession of developmental phases, each of which was thought to build on and subsume the accomplishments of the preceding phases. Consequently, he described the oral phase, the anal phase, and the phallic phase. Thus, the oral phase occupied the first twelve to eighteen months of the infant's life, the anal phase the following period until about age three, and finally the phallic phase from ages three to five.

Initially, erotic activity in the phallic phase is linked with urination. Freud discussed in passing the urethral phase, which was subsequently elaborated by later writers. Freud postulated, however, that in boys, phallic erotic activity was essentially a preliminary stage for adult genital activity. In contrast to the male, whose principal sexual organ remained the penis throughout the course of psychosexual development, the female has two leading erotogenic zones, the clitoris and the vagina. Freud felt that the clitoris was preeminent during the infantile genital period but that erotic primacy after puberty was transmitted to the vagina. It should be noted that recent sexual investigations have cast some doubt on a transition from clitoral to vaginal primacy but that many analysts retain this view on the basis of clinical findings. The question for the moment remains unresolved.

The basic schema offered by Freud of the psychosexual stages was modified and refined through the work of Karl Abraham, one of the most gifted of Freud's followers, who further subdivided the phases of libido development, dividing the oral period into a sucking and biting phase, and the anal phase into a destructive-expulsive (anal sadistic) and a mastering-retaining (anal erotic) phase. Finally, he hypothesized that the phallic period consisted of an earlier phase of partial genital love, which was designated as the true phallic phase, and a later, more mature genital phase.

For each of the stages of psychosexual development, Freud delineated specific erotogenic zones that, when stimulated, gave rise to erotic gratification. Freud suggested that, in addition, there were at least three phases of genital masturbatory activity: during early infancy, at the high point of infantile sexuality in the phallic phase, and again during puberty. During the earliest months of life the genital region was often stimulated as a natural part of parental caretaking activity. Direct masturbatory activity, however—that is, stimulation of the penis in boys and the clitoris in girls—reaches a peak sometime during the phallic phase and continues until the end of the oedipal period. Table A provides a résumé of current, more or less tentative, views on psychosexual development (see appendix).

Theory of the Instincts

When Freud began his investigation into the nature of unconscious drives, he strove consistently to base psychoanalytic theory on a firm biological foundation. Only when this attempt was frustrated, as was apparent in his attempt to formulate a complete physiological theory in the *Project*, did he retreat from this idea. One of the most important measures of this attempt to link psychological and biological phenomena came in the context of Freud's basing his theory of motivation on instincts. As was noted in the previous discussion of instincts, Freud viewed the instincts as a class of borderline concepts that functioned between the mental and organic spheres. Consequently, his use of the term "instinct" is not always consistent because it emphasizes either the psychic or biological aspect of the term in varying degrees in varying contexts. Sometimes, then, libido refers to the somatic process underlying the sexual instinct, and at other times, it refers to the psychological representation itself. Thus, Freud's usage is quite divergent from the Darwinian implications of the term "instinct," which implies innate, inherited, unlearned, and biologically adaptive behavior.

The clearest formulation of the notion of instinct came in Freud's 1915 paper "Instincts and Their Vicissitudes." "Instinct" is used there as a concept that functions between the mental and the somatic realms as a psychic representative of stimuli, which come from the organism and exercise their influence on the mind. They are thus a measure of the demand made on the mind for work as a result of its connection with the body. Although it is immediately clear that this concept plays an essential role in the psychoanalytic understanding of the function of the mind, the concept nonetheless remains somewhat ambiguous. The relationship between psychological and somatic processes is particularly difficult to elucidate. The difficulty is not diminished by simply affirming a conviction of the essential psychosomatic unity of mind and body.

Psychoanalysts are forced, just as Freud was, to limit their theoretical constructs primarily to the psychological aspects of human behavior. Again and again in the course of the development of psychoanalytic thinking, there have been attempts to free psychoanalytic concepts from the cloying involvement with the somatic, biological organism. Most recently, for example, object relations theorists have been demanding that instinctual theory be abandoned as a biological aberration, which was simply a peculiarity of Freud's thinking that only inhibits the development of a more purely psychological science. This is Freud's "as if" again. The problem remains, however, as to whether or not a disembodied psychology can be a psychology of human nature in any real sense. The tension remains in psychoanalytic thinking, and the author only wishes to note here that the tension was inherent in the very beginning of Freud's thinking about instincts and in the ambiguities over the formulation of the concept of instinct, which he was never able to resolve. If at this point the problem of mind versus body, or of instinctual representation versus organismic stimulus, cannot be resolved, at least where the ambiguity persists can be made clear.

Characteristics of the Instincts

In Freud's description of instincts he ascribed to them four principal characteristics: source, impetus, aim, and object. In general the *source* of an instinct refers to the part of the body from which it arises, the biological substratum that gives rise to the organismic stimuli. The source, then, refers to a somatic process that gives rise to stimuli, which are represented in the mental life as drive representations or affects. In the case of libido the stimulus refers to the process or factors that excite a specific erotogenic zone. The *impetus* or pressure is a quantitative-economic concept that refers to the amount of force or energy or demand for work made by the instinctual stimulus. The *aim* is any action directed toward satisfaction or tension release. The aim in every instinct is satisfaction, which can only be obtained by reducing the state of stimulation at the source of the instinct. The *object* is the person or thing that is the target for this satisfaction-seeking action and that enables the instinct to gain satisfaction or discharge the tension and thus gain the instinctual aim of pleasure.

Freud commented that the object was the most variable characteristic of the instinct, because it is only appropriate to the extent that its characteristics make satisfaction possible. At times the subject's own body may serve as an object of an instinct as, for example, in masturbatory activity. Although this early view of the instinctual object long held sway in psychoanalytic thinking, it has come under some serious criticism recently. Considerably more weight is put on the significance of the objects of libidinal attachment, particularly by object relations theorists. Increasingly, it has become apparent that the psychoanalytic concept of instincts is meaningless, unless it includes and derives from a context of object relatedness. Moreover, it cannot be said simply that the objects of infantile drives are the most variable characteristic of the instinct, because attachment to the primary objects, particularly the mothering object, is of the utmost significance developmentally.

Vicissitudes of Infant Sexuality

During infancy and early childhood, erotic sensation emanates for the most part from the mucosal surfaces of a particular body part or organ. Specifically, during the earliest years of life, the mucous membranes of the mouth, anus, or external genitalia are the appropriate primary focus of the child's erotic life. The focus will vary depending on the phase of psychosexual development. Subsequently, the sexual activity in normal adults is dominated by the genital zone. Nonetheless, the pregenital or prephallic erotogenic functioning of the oral and anal zones still retains a place in sexual activity, specifically in preliminary mating activities (or foreplay). Stimulation of such zones elicits preliminary gratification (forepleasure) that precedes coitus. In normal adults who have achieved a level of mature genital potency, the sexual act will culminate in the pleasure (end pleasure) of orgasm.

Part Instincts

Freud described the erotic impulses arising from the pregenital zone as component or part instincts. Thus, kissing, stimulation of the area surrounding the anus, or even biting the love object in the course of lovemaking are examples of activities associated with these part instincts. The activity of component instincts or early genital excitement may undergo displacement, as for example to the eyes in looking and being looked at (scoptophilia), and may consequently be a source of pleasure. Ordinarily, these component instincts undergo repression or persist in a restricted fashion in sexual foreplay. More specifically, young children are characterized by a polymorphous-perverse sexual disposition. Their total sexuality is relatively undifferentiated and encompasses all of the part instincts. In the normal course of development to adult genital maturity, however, these part instincts are presumed to become subordinate to the primacy of the genital region. The failure to achieve genital primacy may result in a variety of forms of pathology. If, for example, the libido becomes too firmly attached to one of the pregenital erotogenic zones, or a single part instinct becomes predominant, a perversion such as fellatio or voyeurism, which under ordinary circumstances would be limited to the preliminary stages of lovemaking, would replace the normal act of sexual intercourse, even to the extent that orgastic satisfaction can be derived from it. The persistent attachment of the sexual instinct to a particular stage of pregenital development is called a "fixation."

Neurosis and Perversion

Freud further discovered that in the psychoneuroses only a limited number of sexual impulses that had been repressed and were responsible for neurotic symptoms were of a "normal kind." Usually, the repressed and pathogenic impulses were the same impulses that were given overt expression in the perversions. He thus regarded the neurosis as the negative of perversions. It seems, however, that the relationship between the psychoneuroses and perversions is not nearly so simple as that. The situation is considerably more complex. For example, even at the current point of its development, Freud's theory cannot account for the fact that in one case a part instinct might be re-pressed and provide the stimulus for neurotic symptom formation, whereas in another case the part instinct may remain overt and domi-nate the individual's sexual activity in the form of a perversion. In other words, although the theory of sexuality included the concept of libidinal fixation, to the extent that it was limited to the description of various potential zones of libidinal stimulation and excitement, it was unable to explain the outcome of fixation in a particular case. The resolution of this problem had to await the development of later parts of the theory, particularly those concerning defense mechanisms, the functions of ego and superego, as well as the nature and role of anxiety in mental functioning.

SIX

Development and Object Relations

CURRENT THEORIES IN psychoanalytic psychiatry have focused increasingly on the importance for later psychopathology of early disturbances in object relationships; that is, a disturbance in the relationship between the child's affect and the significant objects in the environment, particularly the mothering object. Students of development, who emphasize the importance of cultural factors in development, have criticized Freud for setting forth his notions of psychosexual development in a "social vacuum" without taking into account the influence on the child's instinctual development of the adult objects with whom there is contact. The criticism does not seem to be altogether warranted. From his earliest writings on sexual development, Freud incorporated the basic notion of an object relationship as intimately connected to the functioning of the sexual instinct. He considered the aspects of drive discharge and object attachment as closely interwoven aspects of instinctual phenomena. Even from the very beginning of the child's development, Freud regarded the sexual instinct as "anaclitic," in the sense that the child's attachment to the feeding and mothering figure is based on the child's utter physiological dependence on the object. This view is not surprising when considering that the libido theory evolved from Freud's insight, acquired early in his clinical experience, that the sexual fantasies of even adult patients typically centered on early relationships with their parents. In any event, throughout his descriptions of the libidinal phases of development, Freud made constant reference to the significance of children's relationships with crucial figures in their environment. Specifically, he postulated that the choice of a love object in adult life, the love relationship itself, and object relationships in other spheres of interest and activity would depend largely on the nature and quality of the child's object relationships during the earliest years of life.

Lines of Development

An important contribution to the understanding of development was made by Anna Freud in 1965 with her concept of developmental lines. Developmental lines can be traced for any given area of the personality and its functioning. They are equivalent developmental scales that trace the child's gradual growth out of dependent, infantile, cognitively less mature and organized, id- and object-determined attitudes or modes of functioning toward increasingly mature, autonomous, differentiated levels and modes of action that reflect increasing ego mastery over internal and external environments. The developmental level achieved by the child in any area reflects the outcome of complex interactions between drive and ego-superego development, on one hand, and environmental influences, on the other. The developmental line consequently traces the course of interaction among elements of maturation, adaptation, and structuralization.

One of the most important of such developmental lines—even a prototype for other developmental lines—is that which describes the sequence of relationship with objects reaching from primary infantile dependence to young adult independence and self-reliance. Anna Freud describes it in these terms:

1. The biological unity between the mother-infant couple, with the mother's narcissism extending to the child, and the child including the mother in his [or her] internal "narcissistic milieu" (Hoffer), the whole period being further subdivided (according to Margaret Mahler) into the autistic, symbiotic, and separation-individuation phases with significant danger points for developmental disturbances lodged in each individual phase;

2. the part object (Melanie Klein), or need-fulfilling, anaclitic relationship, which is based on the urgency of the child's body needs

and drive derivatives and is intermittent and fluctuating, because object cathexis is sent out under the impact of imperative desires and withdrawn again when satisfaction has been reached;

3. the stage of object constancy, which enables a positive inner image of the object to be maintained, irrespective of either satisfactions or dissatisfactions;

4. the ambivalent relationship of the preoedipal, anal-sadistic stage, characterized by the ego attitudes of clinging, torturing, dominating, and controlling the love objects;

5. the completely object-centered phallic-oedipal phase, characterized by possessiveness of the parent of the opposite sex (or vice versa), jealousy of and rivalry with the parent of the same sex, protectiveness, curiosity, bids of admiration, and exhibitionistic attitudes; in girls a phallic-oedipal (masculine) relationship to the mother preceding the oedipal relationship to the father;

6. the latency period, i.e., the postoedipal lessening of drive urgency and the transfer of libido from the parental figures to contemporaries, community groups, teachers, leaders, impersonal ideals, and aim-inhibited, sublimated interests, with fantasy manifestations giving evidence of disillusionment with and denigration of the parents ("family romance," twin fantasies, etc.);

7. the preadolescent prelude to the "adolescent revolt," i.e., a return to early attitudes and behavior, especially of the part object, need-fulfilling, and ambivalent type;

8. the adolescent struggle around denying, reversing, loosening, and shedding the tie to the infantile objects, defending against pregenitality, and finally establishing genital supremacy with libidinal cathexis transferred to objects of the opposite sex, outside the family. [1965:65–66]

This particular developmental line is particularly useful in the assessment of object relations in various forms of adult psychopathology.

Object Relations during Pregenital Phases of Development

At birth, the infant's responses to external stimulation are relatively diffuse and disorganized. Even so, as recent experimental research on neonates has indicated, the infant is quite responsive to external stimulation, and the patterns of response are quite complex and relatively organized, even shortly after birth. Even neonates of a few hours of age will respond selectively to novel stimuli and will demonstrate re-markable preferences for complex as compared to simple patterns of stimulation. The infant's responses to noxious and pleasurable stimuli are also relatively undifferentiated. Even so, sensations of hunger, cold, and pain give rise to tension and a corresponding need to seek relief from painful stimuli. At the beginning of life, however, the infant is not responding specifically to objects. A certain degree of develop-ment of perceptual and cognitive apparatuses is required, as well as a greater degree of differentiation of sensory impressions and inte-gration of cognitive patterns, before babies are able to differentiate be-tween the impressions belonging to themselves and those derived from external objects. Consequently, observations and inferences based on data derived from the first six months of life must be interpreted in the context of the child's cognitive functioning before self-object differ-entiation.

In these first months of life, human infants are considerably more helpless than any other young mammals. Their helplessness will con-tinue for a longer period of time than in any other species. They cannot survive unless they are cared for, and they cannot achieve relief from the painful disequilibrium of inner physiological states with-out the help of external caretaking objects. Object relationships of the most primitive kind only begin to be established when an infant first begins to grasp this fact of experience. In the beginning, an in-fant cannot distinguish between its own lips and its mother's breasts, nor does an infant initially associate the satiation of painful hunger pangs with the presentation of the extrinsic breast. Because the infant is aware only of its own inner tension and relaxation and is unaware of the external object, the longing for the object exists only to the de-gree that the disturbing stimuli persists and the longing for satiation remains unsatisfied in the absence of the object. When the satisfying object finally appears and the infant's needs are gratified, the longing also disappears.

Oral Phase and Objects

It is this experience of unsatisfied need, together with the expe-rience of frustration in the absence of the breast and need-satisfying release of tension in the presence of the breast, that forms the basis of the infant's first awareness of external objects. The first awareness of an object, then, in the psychological sense, comes from the longing for something that is already familiar, for something that actually gratified needs in the past but is not immediately available in the present. Thus, it is basically the infant's hunger that in the beginning compels the recognition of the outside world. The first primitive reaction to objects, putting them into the mouth, then becomes understandable. This reaction is consistent with the modality of the infant's first recognition of reality, judging reality by oral gratification, that is, whether something will provide relaxation of inner tension and satisfaction (and should thereby be incorporated, swallowed) or whether it will create inner tension and dissatisfaction (and consequently should be spit out).

Early in this interaction the mother has served an important function, that of empathically responding to the infant's inner needs in such a manner as to become involved in a process of mutual regulation, which maintains the homeostatic balance of the infant's physiological needs and processes within tolerable limits. Not only does this process keep the child alive, but it sets a rudimentary pattern of experience within which the child can build the elements of a basic trust that promotes reliance on the benevolence and availability of caretaking objects. Consequently, the mother's administrations and responsiveness to the child help to lay down the most rudimentary and essential foundation for the subsequent development of object relations and the capacity for entering the community of human beings.

As the differentiation between the limits of self and object is gradually established in the child's experience, the mother becomes acknowledged and recognized as the source of gratifying nourishment and, in addition, as the source of the erotogenic pleasure the infant derives from sucking on the breast. In this sense she becomes the first love object. The quality of the child's attachment to this primary object is of the utmost importance. From the oral phase onward, the whole progression in psychosexual development, with its focus on successive erotogenic zones and the emergence of associated component instincts, will reflect the quality of the child's attachment to the crucial figures in the environment, as well as the strength of feelings of love or hate, or both, toward these important persons. If a fundamentally warm, trusting, and affectionate relationship has been established between mother and child during the earliest stages of the child's career, then at least theoretically, the stage will be set for the development of trusting and affectionate relationships with other human objects during the course of life.

It is only recently that any extensive awareness has been developed of the complexities of the oral stage of development and the vicissitudes to which the interaction between mother and child can be exposed. Increasingly, there is a growing awareness of the multiple aspects of the mother's own personality and functioning, which can impede or interfere with the normal pattern of development within the child. The nursing and caretaking interaction with the child can become the focus for a variety of conflicts and pathological influences deriving from disturbances in the mother-child relationship or from the mother's own personal inadequacies or psychopathology.

Aside from the adverse consequences typically associated with maternal rejection or undue frustration of the infant's needs, distortions in the early mother-child relationship may have more subtle, if equally severe, repercussions. The earlier stage of oral eroticism is succeeded by an increase of oral sadistic impulses in the biting phase. Inevitably, the frustration associated with the latter part of the oral period, and particularly with the weaning process, which to the child signifies the imminent loss of gratification and rejection, can evoke biting and cannibalistic impulses toward the object. When such impulses are excessive, as they might be under conditions of maternal rejection or unresponsiveness, they can serve as a prelude for later, more serious impairments of object relations.

A distinction should be made between infants' biological relation to their mothers in this early stage of life and their psychological relation to their mothers. Clearly, from the very beginning of life, even before birth in the child's prenatal dependence on the mother, there is a biological bond between mother and child that satisfies the basic biological and physiological needs of the child. The psychological counterpart of this dependence, however, is not at all evident in the early months of life to external observation and may, in fact, take many months to develop. Although some authors may speak of a primitive emotional bond between mother and child in the first months of life, such an emotional relationship cannot develop before some degree of differentiation between self and object in the child's experience.

One can speak meaningfully at this level of psychological organization of primitive affective responses, of pleasure and unpleasure, which may relate to states of physiological homeostasis. Such reactions are physiologically derived and do not imply awareness of the object as separately existing but, nonetheless, may be regarded as providing the primitive basis for later psychological differentiation and for the emergence of affective ties to the object. In 1939 Hartmann commented in this regard as follows: "[W]e should not assume, from the fact that the child and the environment interact from the outset, that the child is from the beginning psychologically directed toward the object as an object" (1939:52). Thus, there is a distinction to be drawn between the biological "state of adaptedness," or actual relatedness to the object that exists from birth, and the psychological adaptation to the object that follows on structural differentiation and the recognition of the object as separate from the self. This early stage of infantile adaptation has been described as undifferentiated, autistic, or objectless.

Mahler's Autistic Phase

Margaret Mahler's work has been particularly useful in conceptualizing the process of development in terms of the phases of separation-individuation. The first phase of development that Mahler describes is the autistic phase:

> we would propose to distinguish two stages within the phase of primary narcissism (a Freudian concept to which we find it most useful to adhere). During the first few weeks of extrauterine life, a stage of absolute primary narcissism, marked by the infant's lack of awareness of a mothering agent, prevails. This is the stage we have termed *normal autism*. It is followed by a stage of dim awareness that need satisfaction cannot be provided by oneself, but comes from somewhere outside the self. . . .

The task of the autistic phase is the achievement of homeostatic equilibrium of the organism within the new extramural environment, by predominantly somatopsychic physiological mechanisms. [1975:42, 43]

To the external observer, newborn infants seem to relate to their mothers in a condition of unique dependence and responsiveness. This relationship is, however, at least at first, purely biological, based on physiological reflexes and ordered to the fulfillment of basic biological needs. It is only as babies' egos begin to develop, along with the organization of perceptual capacities and memory traces, which allow for the initial differentiation of self and object, that infants can be said to experience something outside of themselves, to which they can relate, as satisfying their inner needs. This dawning awareness of the external object is a most significant state in the psychological development of children and involves not only cognitive and perceptual developments but also goes hand in hand with the organization of rudimentary infantile drives and affects in relation to emerging object experiences.

Freud's view in 1930 of this process is that infants gradually learn to distinguish between their own bodily selves and external objects by the repeated discovery that some sources of stimulus and gratification are always available, whereas others are not. The former become linked with their own bodies, whereas the others are connected with the intermittently appearing and disappearing mother, initially with the mother's breast as a satiating and discomfort-relieving part-object. The pleasure principle demands that sensations of pain or unpleasure be avoided and sensations of pleasure or satiation be sought. In the beginning the sources of unpleasure are attributed to the world outside the self, thus creating what Freud called a "pure pleasure ego."

As the child's experience develops, the maintenance of the pure pleasure ego becomes more difficult as some of the unpleasurable experiences are found to be internally derived, whereas pleasurable experiences are also experienced as originating outside of the self. These early affective experiences in relation to the gratification or frustration of needs are put in the service of building up self- and object-representations as an initial phase of the organization of psychic structures. These representational components, deriving from such affectively toned experiences, are initially organized at the rather crude level of differentiating pleasure from unpleasure. As the child gradually learns to differentiate self from object in this representational sphere, the libidinal attachment to the object is specifically a function of the object's need-satisfying capacity.

Initially, these perceptual organizations may be created in the immediate context of need gratification and cease to function at those points in the infant's experience where need gratification is no longer operative. These early fragmentary experiences of need gratification and their connection with the object are continually reinforced so that they begin to take on a more constant structural organization that keeps them continually available. This increasing differentiation is put in the service of the infant's adaptive needs, and gradually the functional differentiation of the perceptual and affective level becomes increasingly autonomous and is consolidated as a structural acquisition of the infant's emerging ego.

Gradually, as the infant's experience is amplified and reinforced, the attachment to and valuation of the object become relatively independent of the need-gratifying functions of the object. In the classical theory, it is at this point of the emerging experience of and attachment to the object that primary narcissism yields to secondary narcissism. Primary narcissism may be thought of as that infantile state in which the predominant feeling tone of the infant is one of self-contained pleasure. Such a primitive state can exist only before the differentiation of the self and object and their respective representations. Consequently, primary narcissism is not correctly thought of as a cathexis of the self because the self is not yet at this stage structurally organized nor experientially differentiated. At this stage of internal development, there is not yet available a self-representation but, rather, only a qualitative organization of the infant's experience. It is the child's early attachment to the need-satisfying object and the emerging psychological relationship to that object that change the quality of the child's experience and begin to modify primary narcissism.

The emergence of the psychological need-satisfying relationship to the object or part-object occurs during the oral phase of libidinal development. It should be noted, however, that the notion of the oral phase of development and the concepts of need-satisfying relationships are not equivalent. The oral phase is primarily concerned with libidinal development and stresses the predominance of the oral zone as the main erotogenic zone. The concept of need-satisfying relationship, however, is not concerned directly with issues of drive development but, rather, with the characteristics of object involvement and object relationship.

In writing of this need-satisfying relationship, Anna Freud emphasizes that the relationship at this stage is intermittent, existing only at times of need and ceasing to exist once the needs are gratified: "object cathexis is sent out under the impact of imperative desires, and withdrawn again when satisfaction has been reached" (1965:65). In other words, the mother is perceived only in terms of her capacity to satisfy the infant's needs and not as a whole, separately existing object in her own right. This phase of development corresponds to Mahler's symbiotic phase (2 to 6 months) in which the child's awareness of the mother exists only as a need-satisfying quasi extension of the child's own self.

Mahler's Symbiotic Phase

According to Mahler and associates, this awareness signals the beginning of normal symbiosis "in which the infant behaves and functions as though he and his mother were an omnipotent system—a dual unity within one common boundary" (1975:44). The symbiotic phase, also according to Mahler and associates, is described in the following terms:

> The essential feature of symbiosis is hallucinatory or delusional somatopsychic *omnipotent* fusion with the representation of the mother and, in particular, the delusion of a common boundary between two physically separate individuals. This is the mechanism to which the ego regresses in cases of the most severe disturbance of individuation and psychotic disorganization, which Mahler (1952) has described as "symbiotic child psychosis."
>
> In the human species, the function of and the equipment for self-preservation are atrophied. The rudimentary (not yet functional) ego in the newborn baby and the young infant has to be complemented by the emotional rapport of the mother's nursing care, a kind of social symbiosis. It is within this matrix of physiological and sociobiological dependency on the mother

that the structural differentiation takes place which leads to the individual's organization for adaptation: the functioning ego. [1975:45]

These boundaries become temporarily differentiated only in the state of "affect hunger" but disappear again as a result of need gratification. Only gradually does the child form more stable part-images of the mother, such as breasts, face, or hands. Consequently, in 1972 Edgcumbe and Burgner concluded that

> the crucial distinguishing characteristic of the stage of need satisfaction (variously referred to also as the anaclytic or symbiotic phase) is that the object is recognized as separate from the self only at moments of need; once the need is satisfied, we assume that—from the infant's (subjective) point of view—the object then ceases to exist until a need arises again. In other terms, cathexis is withdrawn from the object. Moreover, from the infant's point of view, the relationship is not to a specific object (or part-object) but rather to the *function* of having the need satisfied and to the accompanying pleasure afforded by the object in fulfilling that function. [1972:298–299]

It is only when the specific object—that is, the whole object—becomes as important to the child as the need-satisfying function that it performs that one can regard the child's development as moving beyond the level of need-satisfying relationships toward the attainment of object constancy.

Although it is clear that the oral phase of libidinal development and need-satisfying relationships are not synonymous, there is a tendency to use the terms with overlapping significance. They should be kept distinct. The need-satisfying relationship is specifically a mode or quality of interaction in which it is the object's need-satisfying functions that assume prime importance to the subject. In contrast, demanding, greedy, or passive and dependent attitudes toward the object are often described as "oral." The conflation of "oral" with "need-satisfying" can thus give rise to considerable confusion, particularly where certain forms of character traits or other aspects of drive and ego organization may be described as oral to the extent that they represent persistent formations from the oral phase of drive development. Such developmental characteristics, however, may not imply the persistence of need-gratifying relationships at all.

To the extent that many of the behaviors toward objects represent clinging, egocentric, demanding, greedy, or selfish forms of behavior in relation to objects, they can be described as need-gratifying. Such behaviors, however, may be closely involved with underlying needs to satisfy narcissistic or even sexual drive pressures that may derive from multiple levels of development. This context of reference is quite different from that implied by the developmental arrest or regression to a phase of need-satisfying relationships. This latter phenomenon is observed rarely even in psychotic or borderline children. Consequently, care should be taken in the use of such terms as to what is implied specifically with reference to the quality of object relationships and their developmental implications.

A useful caution with respect to such concepts is that, although psychological functioning can begin in rudimentary ways shortly after birth or even to some degree at birth, the same cannot be said of the organization of psychological relationships. The emergence of such relationships requires the forming of at least rudimentary representation of the external environment as external. The organization of the infant's psychological capacities and differentiating structures, adequate to allow even primitive representation of need-gratifying objects, probably requires several months and may only begin to emerge by about the third month of life. Even then the organization of these capacities remains intermittent and unstable and is closely tied to states of need gratification. Nonetheless, they provide the beginnings of psychological relationships to objects and the rudimentary organization of these basic capacities.

Thus, the presence of certain identifiable perceptual capacities of primary autonomy cannot be regarded as proof that other aspects of psychic functioning have been elaborated. Even at birth the child seems capable of organizing primitive perceptual formations that rapidly become more complex and sophisticated. The presence, however, of such perceptual structures does not imply that they are ipso facto used by the infant in a context of psychological relationship to an object. The hungry infant may grow quiet and show signs of responding to the stimuli associated with feeding, but this by no means implies the capability of recognizing the mother as a separate object or the capability of maintaining any connection or relationship with her once the hunger need has been satisfied. Even the development of "stranger anxiety" in the child at eight months does not necessarily indicate the establishment of such a constant relationship to the mother. It suggests no more than that the child has begun to distinguish between objects and has begun to invest in the representation of the mother, but this does not yet imply that there is any cathectic attachment to or valuation of the mother as a whole person beyond her ability or function as satisfying certain specific needs.

Thus, it is useful to distinguish between need satisfaction as a stage of development in object relationships, related to but not synonymous with the oral phase of libidinal development, and need satisfaction as a determinant in object relationships at every level of development. The satisfaction of various kinds of psychological needs continues to play a role at all levels of object relatedness, but the satisfaction of such needs cannot be used as a distinguishing characteristic of the specific stage of need-satisfying object relationships. As objects become increasingly differentiated in the child's experience, their representations achieve increasing psychological complexity and value in a context of increasingly complex and subtle needs for a variety of input from objects. The development of object constancy implies a constant relationship to a specific object, but within that relationship the wish for satisfaction of needs and the actual satisfaction of those needs may be a significant component of the object relationship.

Anal Phase and Objects

During the oral stage of the development, the infant's role is not altogether passive because of being caught up in a process of mutual interaction, by reason of which there is a contribution to eliciting certain responses from the mother. The activity, however, is more or less automatic and dependent on such physiological factors as level of activity, irritability, or responsiveness to stimuli. Generally speaking, however, the infant's control over the mother's feeding responses is relatively limited. Consequently, the primary onus remains on the mother to gratify or frustrate the demands of the infant.

In the transition to the anal period, however, this picture changes significantly. The child acquires a greater degree of control over behavior and particularly over sphincter function. Moreover, for the first time during this period the demand is placed on the child to relinquish some aspect of freedom in that there is an expectation to accede to the parental demand that the toilet be used for evacuation of feces and urine. However, the primary aim of anal eroticism is the enjoyment of the pleasurable sensation of excretion. Somewhat later the stimulation of the anal mucosa through retention of the fecal mass may become a source of even more intense pleasure. Nonetheless, at this stage of development the demand is placed on the child to regulate gratification, to surrender some portion of the gratification at the parent's wish, or to delay the gratification according to a schedule established by the parent's wishes. It can be readily seen that one of the important aspects of the anal period, therefore, is that it sets the stage for a contest of wills over when, how, and on what terms the child will achieve gratification.

The connection between anal and sadistic drives may be attributed to two factors. First, the feces themselves become the object of the first anal-sadistic activity. The pinching off and expulsion of the fecal mass is perceived as a sadistic act. Subsequently, the child can begin to treat objects as the feces were previously treated. The sense of social power evolving from sphincter control provides the second sadistic element: in training for cleanliness, the child exerts power over the mother by means of control over evacuatory functions. The child can exert power over her by yielding and giving up the fecal mass or by refusing to yield and withholding the fecal mass. The struggle can easily become one of who has whose way, and the child's sense of sphincter control gives a sense of power that can easily be threatened. If attempts to stubbornly withhold are excessively punished or the loss of control is excessively shamed, the child may regress to more primitive and oral patterns of relating to the mother.

The first anal strivings are autoerotic. Pleasurable elimination and later pleasurable retention do not require any outside help from an object. Thus, at this stage of development, defecation is accompanied by a sense of omnipotence, and the feces, which are the agency of this pleasure, become a libidinal object. The feces are invested with a high cathexis of narcissistic libido. Although they become external in the act of defecation, they have a high degree of narcissistic cathexis because they represent an object that was once part of one's own body. The loss of highly cathected, powerful, narcissistically invested material is threatening to the child, who wishes to retain or regain the lost feces to restore the narcissistic equilibrium. In this way the feces become an ambivalently loved object; that is, they are loved and retained or desired, on one hand, or they are hated, "pinched off," and expelled, on the other.

Such ministrations of the mother as diaper changes during this period are also associated with pleasurable anal sensations. The quality of maternal care, in combination with conflicts surrounding toilet training, can alter the direction of object strivings. The combination of gratifying and punitive aspects of this interaction can contribute and intensify the ambivalent strivings. There is a tendency for the attitudes toward feces to be displaced toward objects. For example, consider the obsessive-compulsive neurotic individual. The compulsive neatness so characteristic of this syndrome reflects the patient's regression to the anal pregenital phase of development and expresses a wish to dominate. Such individuals exert power over things and people and force them into rigid and pedantic systems. At the same time, this neurotic's feelings are characterized by the ambivalence of the anal strivings—that is, the tendency that wants to control and retain the object—together with the desire to expel and destroy it. The ambivalence so characteristic of the obsessive person is derived from the anal eroticism, which reflects itself in the child's developmental tendency to treat feces in a contradictory manner. The child alternately expels them from the body and retains them as a loved object.

It can be said that in a sense ambivalence is universal and that there is no object relationship of any significance or duration that does not contain elements of both love and hate. When, however, the elements of the ambivalence are intensified and neurotically distorted, the conflict is usually resolved by the repression of one or other aspect of the ambivalence. It is usually the hateful and destructive impulses toward the object that are repressed, particularly in obsessive-compulsive conditions; however, the positive affect may also be repressed, as is often seen in paranoid conditions.

Mahler's Separation and Individuation

During this period, the process of separation and individuation continues to evolve. Through that process the child with effort gradually is differentiated out of the symbiotic matrix. The first behavioral signs of such differentiation seem to arise at about four or five months of age, at the high point of the symbiotic period. The first stage of this process of differentiation is described as "hatching" from the symbiotic orbit:

> In other words, the infant's attention, which during the first months of symbiosis was in large part *inwardly* directed, or focused in a coenesthetic vague way *within the symbiotic orbit,* gradually expands through the coming into being of outwardly directed perceptual activity during the child's increasing periods of wakefulness. This is a change of degree rather than of kind, for during the symbiotic stage the child has certainly been highly attentive to the mothering figure. But gradually that attention is combined with a growing store of memories of mother's comings and goings, of "good" and "bad" experiences; the latter were altogether unrelievable by the self, but could be "confidently expected" to be relieved by mother's ministrations. [Mahler 1975:53–54]

As the child's differentiation and separation from the mother gradually increases, there is a move to the second or "practicing" subphase of separation and individuation. The practicing period can be usefully divided into an early practicing period and a practicing period proper. The early practicing phase begins with the infant's earliest ability to move physically away from the mother by locomotion; that is, crawling, creeping, climbing, and resuming an upright sitting position. Moving away from the safe protective orbit of the mother has its risks and uncertainties, however. In the early practicing phase there is frequently a pattern of visually "checking back to mother" or even crawling or paddling back to her to touch or hold on as a form of "emotional refueling."

The practicing period proper is characterized by the attainment of free upright locomotion. It is marked by three interrelated developments that contribute to the continuing process of separation and individuation. These are (1) the rapid bodily differentiation from the mother, (2) the establishment of a specific bond with her, and (3) the growth and functioning of autonomous ego-apparatuses in close connection and dependence on the mothering figure. Mahler and associates comment:

> With the spurt in autonomous functions, such as cognition, but especially upright locomotion, the "love affair with the world" (Greenacre, 1957) begins. The toddler takes the greatest step in human individuation. He walks freely with upright posture. Thus, the plane of his vision changes; from an entirely new vantage point he finds unexpected and changing perspectives, pleasures, and frustrations. There is a new visual level that the upright, bipedal position affords. [1975:70–71]

As this testing of the freedom of individuation proceeds, the child enters the third subphase, that of rapprochement, by about the middle of the second year.

> He now becomes more and more aware, and makes greater and greater use, of his physical separateness. However, side by side with the growth of his cognitive faculties and the increasing differentiation of his emotional life, there is also a noticeable waning of his previous imperviousness to frustration, as well as a diminution of what has been a relative obliviousness to his mother's presence. Increased separation anxiety can be observed: at first this consists mainly of fear of object loss, which is to be inferred from many of the child's behaviors. The relative lack of concern about the mother's presence that was characteristic of the practicing subphase is now replaced by seemingly constant concern with the mother's whereabouts, as well as by active approach behavior. As the toddler's *awareness* of separateness grows—stimulated by his maturationally acquired ability to move away physically from his mother and by his cognitive growth—he seems to have an increased need, a wish for mother to share with him every one of his new skills and experiences, as well as a great need for the object's love. [Mahler 1975:76–77]

The crisis in the rapprochement phase is particularly that of separation anxiety. The child's wishes and desires to be separate, autonomous, and omnipotent are tempered by an increasing awareness of the need for and dependence on the mother. Ambivalence is characteristic of the middle phase of the rapprochement subphase. There is a tension between the child's need to use the mother as a personal extension, as having her magically fulfill wishes, and the realization that, with the child's increasing separateness, she becomes less available and more distant. Thus, the mother's availability and the reassurance of her continuing love and support become all the more important.

As the developments of the rapprochement phase are gradually realized, the child enters the fourth and final phase of separation and individuation; namely, the phase of consolidation of individuality and the beginnings of emotional object constancy. At this stage there are significant developments in the structuralization and integration of the ego, as well as definite signs of internalization of parental demands reflecting the development of superego precursors. The development of emotional object constancy depends on the gradual internalization of a constant, well-integrated, and positive inner image of the mother.

Phallic Phase and Objects

The passage from the anal phase to the phallic phase marks not only the transition from the preoedipal to the beginnings of the oedipal level of development, but also marks the completion of the work of separation-individuation and, in the normal course of development, the achievement of object constancy.

The attainment of object constancy marks a transition from the stage of need-satisfying relationships to a more mature psychological involvement with objects. Object constancy implies a capacity to differentiate between objects and to maintain a meaningful relationship with one specific object whether needs are being satisfied or not. Object constancy in the psychoanalytic sense must be distinguished from perceptual object constancy as described, for example, by Piaget. Perceptual constancy, envisioned by Piaget as developing between ages five to eighteen months, implies the ability to differentiate between self and external objects, to organize relatively stable representations of both self and object, and finally, to maintain a perceptual image of the object in its absence. This is only one component of libidinal constancy in the psychoanalytic sense. Such object constancy also implies the stability of object cathexis and specifically the capacity to maintain positive emotional attachments to a particular object in the face of frustration of needs and wishes in regard to that object. This achievement also implies the capacity to tolerate ambivalent feelings toward the object and the capacity to value that object for qualities that it possesses over and beyond the functions that it may serve in satisfying needs and in gratifying drives.

Consequently, the achievement of object constancy implies a complex and significant internal development in the subject, particularly having to do with the consolidation of relatively autonomous ego functions and their harmonious integration with drive derivatives. In this connection, separation anxiety suggests the beginning of the establishment of a libidinal object and the discrimination of that object from other humans. Similarly, the fear of loss of the love object and the fear of losing the love of that object are also related to the dynamics of object constancy. In 1950 Ernst Kris commented in this regard:

> When in 1926 Freud entered into the discussion of typical danger situations to which the human child is exposed, he distinguished two—the two most archaic ones—which have a direct bearing on object relations: the danger of losing the love object and the danger of losing the object's love. The first represents the anaclytic needs; the second, the more integrated relationship to a permanent, personalized love object that can no longer easily be replaced. . . . Quite obviously, what is true of any other division into phases in the child's life is also true of this distinction: there are not only fluctuations from one type of object relation to the other, older one, but the two types normally overlap. The fear of object loss never quite disappears; the fear of loss of love adds a new dimension to a child's life and with it a new vulnerability. [1975:65–66]

It should be noted that the achievement of libidinal object constancy is a developmental attainment that is never superseded or outgrown but, rather, is expanded and amplified in the normal course of development. All subsequent developmental progress in the capacity for object relationships is really a deepening and extending of this original capacity for object constancy. Moreover, the developmental failure to establish object constancy will have severe implications for all areas of psychic functioning, including drives, ego functions, affective experience, and the capacity for human relationships.

To summarize, it can be said that the notion of object constancy implies the involvement of a number of specific elements that are central to the further emergence of the meaningful capacity for relationships with objects. These elements include perceptual object constancy; the capacity to maintain drive attachment to a specific object whether it is present or not; the capacity to tolerate both loving and hostile feelings toward the same object or to maintain a loving relationship with the object in the face of hostile and destructive impulses; the capacity to maintain significant emotional attachment to a single specific object; and finally, the capacity to value the object for qualities and attributes that it possesses in itself, in virtue of its own uniqueness as individually and separately existing, and as independent of any need-satisfying function it may serve.

Thus, although the concept of libidinal object attachment and object constancy provides the basic components for the emergence of significant object relationships in adult life, it contains the elements by implication that lead to a concept of object relationships that transcends merely libidinal implications. Consequently, it would seem to be useful both theoretically and clinically to distinguish between a libidinal object and a love object. Although the libidinal object has primary reference to the connection with libidinal drive organization, it primarily is concerned with diverse images of the object that may satisfy various drive needs and their associated states of libidinal satisfaction (pleasure) or dissatisfaction (unpleasure). By way of contrast, the love object implies an added dimension of the object for which it becomes valued over and above its need-satisfying functions. Consequently, the notion of a love object can be taken as transcending the levels of libidinal drive organization and their satisfaction. This consideration applies with equal force to genital drive organization, as well as to more specifically pregenital and characteristically need-satisfying kinds of relationships. Thus, the concept of a mutually satisfying, reciprocally rewarding love relationship transcends the limits of libidinal attachment, even at the genital level. Although such a mature love relationship must be responsive to a wide variety of human needs in both partners, including libidinal needs, the regard and valuation of the love object are neither limited to nor wholly determined by those needs and their satisfaction. One can thus conceive of meaningful love relationships in which such needs are in some degree frustrated or denied, just as one can conceive of libidinal relationships that do not reach a level of love relationships. The libidinal object is not synonymous with the love object.

Oedipus Complex

In the normal course of development, the so-called pregenital phases are primarily autoerotic. The primary gratification is derived from stimulation of erotogenic zones, while the object forms a significant, although secondary and instrumental, role. A fundamental shift begins to take place in the phallic phase in which the phallus becomes the primary erotogenous zone for both sexes, thus laying a foundation for and initiating a shift of libidinal motivation and intention in the direction of objects. The phallic phase sets the stage for the fundamental task of finding a love object, a dynamic that moves to another level of progression in establishing the genital love relations of the oedipal period, and beyond to more mature object choices and love relationships. The phallic period is also a critical phase of development for the budding formation of the child's own sense of gender identity—as decisively male or female—based on the child's discovery and realization of the significance of anatomical sexual differences. The events associated with the phallic phase also set the stage for the developmental predisposition to later psychoneuroses. Freud used the term "Oedipus complex" to refer to the intense love relationships—together with their associated rivalries, hostilities, and emerging identifications—formed during this period between the child and parents.

Another significant dimension of the entrance onto the phallic stage is that in the pregenital periods the child's relationships have been based primarily on one-to-one relationships with each parent, separately and individually. With regard to both mother and father, in the context of these separate dyadic relationships, the child has worked out such important aspects of interpersonal relating as trust, dependency, autonomy, and, to a certain extent, initiative. As the child emerges into the oedipal period, however, a new level is achieved in the complexity of object relationships in that the child's involvement with the parents is now specifically triadic.

Accompanying this important developmental step from a dyadic to a triadic level of involvement, there are other significant factors; namely, an increased capacity for differentiation between internal and external reality and an increased capacity to tolerate the anxiety of the oedipal involvement. Consequently, the Oedipus complex represents the climax of the development of infantile sexuality. The transition from oral eroticism, through anal eroticism, to genitality, and the various associated stages in the development of object relations, from need gratification, through the emergence of object constancy and simple one-to-one dependency, to the triadic oedipal situation, culminate in the oedipal strivings. An overcoming of these strivings, which can then be replaced in the reworking of adolescence by a more mature and adult sexuality, is a prerequisite for normal development. Conversely, the psychoneuroses are specifically characterized by an unconscious fixation at the phallic phase and an unconscious clinging to oedipal attachments.

The Oedipus complex evolves during the period extending from the third to the fifth year in children of both sexes. There is some discrepancy between the sexes in the pattern of development. Freud explained the nature of this discrepancy in terms of genital differences. Under normal circumstances, he felt, for boys the oedipal situation was resolved by the castration complex. Specifically, the boy had to give up his strivings for his mother because of the threat of castration—castration anxiety. By way of contrast, the Oedipus complex in girls is evoked by reason of the castration complex. Unlike the boy, the little girl is already castrated, and as a result, she turns to her father as the bearer of the penis, out of a sense of disappointment over her own lack of a penis. The little girl is more threatened by a loss of love than by actual castration fears.

Castration Complex

In boys, the development of object relations is relatively less complex than for girls, because the boy remains attached to his first love object, the mother. The primitive object choice of the primary love object, which develops in response to the mother's gratification of the infant's basic needs, takes the same direction as the pattern of object choice that will take place in response to opposite-sex objects in later life experience. In the phallic period, in addition to the child's attachment to and interest in the mother as a source of nourishment, he develops a strong erotic interest in her and a concomitant desire to possess her exclusively and sexually. These feelings usually become manifest at about age three and reach a climax at ages four or five.

With the appearance of the oedipal involvement, the boy begins to show his loving attachment to his mother almost as a little lover might—wanting to touch her, trying to get in bed with her, proposing marriage, expressing wishes to replace his father, and devising opportunities to see her naked or undressed. Competition from siblings for mother's affection and attention is intolerable. Above all, however, the little lover wants to eliminate his arch rival—mother's husband and his father. His wishes may involve not merely displacing or superseding father in mother's affection but eliminating him altogether. The child understandably anticipates retaliation for his aggressive wishes toward his father, and these expectations in turn give rise to a severe anxiety.

Specifically, he begins to feel that his sexual interest in his mother will be punished by removal of his penis. Freud identified this idea of mutilation of the male organ in retaliation for incestuous wishes as the "castration complex." He suggested further, in 1924 in "The Dissolution of the Oedipus Complex," that in the phallic period the narcissistic fear of injury to the penis is actually stronger than the erotic attachment to the mother. Any gratification of the boy's passionate love would thus endanger his penis and threaten him with severe narcissistic loss. Confronted with this threat of castration and the anxiety related to it, the boy must finally renounce his oedipal love for his mother. In renouncing his oedipal attachments and his oedipal ambitions, the boy thus identifies with the father and consequently internalizes the father's prohibitions and restraints. In effect, the castration complex is internalized, thus freeing the child from the threat of external authority and retaliation, until such time as the internalization can be reexternalized under the regressive influence of puberty.

This somewhat simplified picture of the resolution of the Oedipus complex is considerably more complex in the actual course of development. Usually the boy's love for his mother remains a dominant force during the period of infantile sexual development. It is known, however, that love is not free of some admixture of hostility and that the child's relationship with both parents is to some degree ambivalent. The boy also loves his father, and at times when he has been frustrated by his mother, he may hate her and turn from her to seek affection from his father. Undoubtedly, to some degree he both loves and hates both his parents at the same time. In addition, Freud's postulation of an essentially bisexual basis of the nature of the libido complicates matters further. On the one hand, the boy wants to possess his mother and kill the hated father-rival. On the other hand, he also loves his father and seeks approval and affection from him, whereas he often reacts to his mother with hostility, particularly when her demands on her husband interfere with the exclusiveness of the father-son relationship. The "negative Oedipus complex" refers to those situations where the boy's love for his father predominates over the love of the mother, and the mother is relatively hated as a disturbing element in this relationship.

Under certain circumstances, the reversal of the typical oedipal triangle may have serious implications for the child's future development. Homosexual development, for example, is often characterized by an unsatisfied longing for closeness with the father and a strong identification with the mother, derived from an unresolved, negative oedipal involvement. It must be emphasized that the negative Oedipus complex is normally present to some degree along with its positive counterpart in normal and healthy development. The point is that under normal conditions these conflicting feelings are able to coexist and can be integrated in a mature pattern of identifications without provoking undue conflict.

The Girl's Situation

Understanding of the little girl's more complex oedipal involvement was a later development. Because it could not be regarded as equivalent to the boy's development, it raised a number of questions that proved to be more difficult. Freud's views had to be elaborated and clarified by the researches of subsequent psychoanalysts, particularly Helene Deutsch, Ruth Mack Brunswick, and Jeanne Lampl-de Groot. Similar to the little boy, the little girl forms an initial attachment to the mother as a primary love object and source of fulfillment for vital needs. For the little boy, the mother remains the love object throughout his development, but the little girl is faced with the task of shifting this primary attachment from the mother to the father to prepare herself for her future sexual role. Freud was basically concerned with elucidating the factors that influenced the little girl to give up her preoedipal attachment to the mother and to form the normal oedipal attachment to the father. A secondary question had to do with the factors that led to the dissolution and resolution of the Oedipus complex in the girl, so that the paternal attachment and the maternal identification would be the basis for adult sexual adjustment.

The girl's renunciation of her preoedipal attachment to the mother could not be satisfactorily explained as the result of ambivalent or aggressive characteristics of the mother-child relationship, for similar elements would influence the relationship between boys and the mother figure. Freud attributed the crucial precipitating factor to the anatomical differences between the sexes—specifically the girl's discovery of the lack of a penis during the phallic period. Up to this point, exclusive of constitutional differences and depending on the variations in parental attitudes in the treatment of a daughter in comparison to a son, the little girl's development parallels that of the little boy.

Fundamental differences, however, emerge when she discovers during the phallic period that her clitoris is inferior to the male counterpart, the penis. The typical reaction of the little girl to this discovery is an intense sense of loss, narcissistic injury, and envy of the male penis. At this point the little girl's attitude to the mother changes. The mother had previously been the object of love, but now she is held responsible for bringing the little girl into the world with inferior genital equipment. The hostility can be so intense that it may persist and color her future relationship to the mother. With the further discovery that the mother also lacks the vital penis, the child's hatred and devaluation of the mother becomes even more profound. In a desperate attempt to compensate for her "inadequacy," the little girl then turns to her father in the vain hope that he will give her a penis, or a baby in place of the missing penis.

The second focus of Freud's concern was on the factors that lead to dissolution of the Oedipus complex in girls. The little girl's sexual love for her father and her hope for a penis-child from him undergo a gradual diminution as a result of her continuing disappointment and frustration. The wish to be loved by her father may foster an identification with mother, whom father loves and to whom he gives children. The threat to the little girl is not the loss of a physical organ, as it is for the little boy, but rather a loss of love—at the first level, from the father who is the object of her attachment and, at a deeper and more infantile level, from the mother as well. Ultimately, the little girl must renounce her father to reattach her libido to a suitable, nonincestuous love object.

Obviously, the Freudian model of feminine psychosexual development has undergone, and is currently undergoing, considerable revision. The charge has been made, and with some justification, that masculine phallic-oedipal development was the primary model in Freud's thinking and that feminine development was viewed as defective in consequence. Freud saw women typically as basically masochistic, weak, dependent, and lacking in conviction, strength of character, and moral fiber. He thought these defects were the result of failure in the oedipal identification with the phallic father because of feminine castration. The resulting internalization of aggression was both constitutionally determined and culturally reinforced.

These concepts must now be regarded as obsolete. Freud's hypotheses of a passive female libido, arrest in ego development, incapacity for sublimation, and superego deficiencies in women are outdated and inadequate. Differences in male and female ego and superego development may be defined, but there are no grounds for judging one to be superior or inferior to the other. They are simply different. As Blum observed in 1976:

> Female development cannot be described in a simple reductionism and overgeneralization. Femininity cannot be predominantly derived from a primary masculinity, disappointed maleness, masochistic resignation to fantasied inferiority, or compensation for fantasied castration and narcissistic injury. Castration reactions and penis envy contribute to feminine character, but penis envy is not the major determinant of femininity. [1976:188]

The adequate conceptualization and understanding of feminine psychology and its development are still very much in process. There is much that is poorly understood and much more that is hardly understood at all. Freud's views in this area cannot be simply jettisoned, because they served and still serve as important signposts along a difficult road. Current research has given partial support to and convincing refutation of his ideas. What is called for is scientific evaluation and theoretical reformulation and modification, rather than rejection. Freud's views will serve better if they are taken as heuristic and tentative formulations, rather than as apodictic postulates. They can be tested, revised, reshaped, and adapted to fit the current realities of feminine psychological functioning. It is not at all clear, in all this, that Freud was so much wrong; he may have simply expressed what he was able to observe in the women of his time and culture. Times change, however, and the culture and the place of women in it has changed and is changing. To that extent, women are different, and much of their psychology is different too. Psychoanalytic understanding must inevitably lag behind these changing patterns of psychological experience, but a new view of feminine development is gradually emerging.

Significance of the Oedipus Complex
As was mentioned, Freud regarded the Oedipus complex as the nucleus for the development of later neuroses and symptom formations. Furthermore, the various admixtures of libidinal fixations, object attachments, and identifications with which the child emerges from the oedipal situation exert a profound influence on the development of character and personality. The introjections accompanying the resolution of oedipal fixations provide the nucleus for the emerging superego.

This whole area is a focus of current concern in psychoanalytically oriented psychiatry. As such, as the child emerges into latency, the processes enabling the resolution of the oedipal situation clearly merit more detailed discussion than has been provided here. These processes are intimately connected with the development of the psychic apparatus and its structural components. Their discussion will be deferred, therefore, to "The Superego" in chapter 9, which is devoted specifically to these areas of psychoanalytic theory. It should be emphasized here, however, that with puberty and the onset of adolescence, there is a resurgence of incestuous oedipal feelings in both sexes so that the task of separating libidinal attachments from parental figures and forming new, more appropriate adult, nonincestuous object attachments to suitable love objects becomes a critical task of the adolescent period. Finally, in young adulthood, with the advent of the biological reality of parenthood, both father and mother each reexperience elements of their own infantile oedipal involvement in their relationships to and identifications with their own children.

Erikson's Epigenetic Sequence:
Instinctual Zones and Modes of Ego Development

Erik Erikson made a major contribution to the psychoanalytic concept of development in his study of the relationship between instinctual zones and the development of specific modalities of ego functioning. Erikson's theory ingeniously links aspects of ego development with the epigenetic timetable of instinctual development.

Erikson postulates a parallel relationship between specific phases of ego or psychosocial development and specific phases of libidinal development. During libidinal development, particular erotogenic zones become the loci of stimulation for the development of particular modalities of ego functioning. The relationship between zones of instinctual stimulation and their corresponding modalities of ego functioning are easily specifiable in the pregenital levels of development, but Erikson projects this basic relationship and extends it to the limits of the life cycle.

Thus, the first modality of development is related to the development in the oral phase, specifically to the stimulus qualities of the oral zone. This early stage is called the oral-respiratory-sensory stage, and it is dominated by the first oral-incorporative mode, which involves the modality of "taking in." This dominant modality is extended to include the whole skin surface and the sense organs, which also become receptive and increasingly hungry for proper stimulation. Other auxiliary modes are also operative, including a second oral-incorporative (biting) mode, an oral-retentive mode, an oral-eliminative mode, and finally, an oral-intrusive mode. These modes become variably important according to individual temperament but remain subordinated to the first incorporative mode unless the mutual regulation of the oral zone with the providing breast of the mother is disturbed, either by a loss of inner control in the infant or a defect in reciprocal and responsive nurturing behavior on the part of the mother. The emphasis in this stage of development is placed on the modalities of "getting," "getting what is given," thus laying the necessary ego groundwork for "getting to be a giver."

The second stage, also focused on the oral zone, is marked by a biting modality because of the development of the teeth. This phase is marked by the development of interpersonal patterns, which center in the social modality of "taking" and "holding" onto things. Thus, incorporation by biting dominates the oral zone at this stage, and the child's libido moves on to endow with power a second organ mode, which leads to the integration of the new social modality, taking. The interplay of zones and modalities, which characterize this complex oral stage of development, forms the springs of a basic sense of "trust" or, conversely, of a basic sense of "mistrust" that remain the basic elements in the most fundamental nuclear conflict in the development of personality.

Similarly, with the advent of the anal-urethral-muscular stage, the "retentive" and "eliminative" modes become established. The extension and generalization of these modes over the whole of the developing muscular system enable the 18- to 24-month-old child to gain some form of self-control in the matter of conflicting impulses, such as "letting-go" and "holding-on." Where this control is disturbed by developmental defects in the anal-urethral sphere, a fixation on the modalities of retention or elimination can be established that can lead to a variety of disturbances in the zone itself (spastic), in the muscle system (flabbiness or rigidity), in obsessional fantasy (paranoid fears), and in social spheres (attempts at controlling the environment by compulsive routinization). The second nuclear conflict, which is derived from the development of these modalities related to the urethral-anal-muscular zones, has to do with the establishment of a basic "autonomy" or, conversely, the establishment of a basic sense of "shame" or "doubt."

Erikson laid out a program of ego development that reached from birth to death: The individual passed through the phases of the life cycle by meeting and resolving a series of developmental psychosocial crises. In the earliest stage of infancy, at the mother's breast, the child developed either a sense of basic trust or a sense of mistrust. In later infancy the child had to achieve a sense of autonomy or, failing that, there would be left some degree of shame and doubt. In early childhood the child developed a sense of initiative, hopefully without guilt. In latency the issue was a sense of industry without a sense of inferiority. The adolescent crisis was the crystallization of the residues of preceding crises into a more or less definitive sense of personal identity, as opposed to a diffusion of identity and a confusion of roles. For the young adult the question was the development of a sense of intimacy, rather than isolation. For the older adult the issue was generativity, as a concern for establishing and guiding the next generation. Finally, in the twilight of life, the crisis to be resolved is that of ego integrity in the face of ultimate despair.

These eight phases of the life cycle and their respective crises accomplished several things. First, they made it clear that ego development was open-ended and never finished. The child's capacity to successfully resolve any one developmental crisis depended on the degree of resolution of the preceding crises. One could form a mature and integral sense of identity only to the extent that one had achieved a meaningful sense of trust, autonomy, initiative, and industry. Successful resolution at any level laid the foundation for engaging in the next developmental crisis. Second, they clarified the relation between the various phases of development and earlier phases of libidinal development. The latter had been the basic contribution of earlier efforts of psychoanalysis, but Erikson's developmental schema gave a better understanding of the way in which earlier libidinal developmental residues were carried along in the course of growth and were built into later developmental efforts of the ego. Psychoanalysis had not previously had the conceptual tools to deal with this problem, particularly in regard to the postadolescent phases of the life cycle. Finally, Erikson's treatment of these crises as specifically psychosocial brought into focus the fact that the development of the ego was not merely a matter of intrapsychic vicissitudes dealing with the economics of inner psychic energies. It was that, certainly, but it was also a matter of the interaction and "mutual regulation" between the developing human organism and significant persons in its environment. Even more strikingly, it is a matter of mutual regulation evolving between the growing child and the culture and traditions of society. Erikson has made the sociocultural influence an integral part of the developmental matrix out of which the personality emerges.

Trust versus Mistrust

The crisis of trust versus mistrust is the first psychosocial crisis the infant must face. It takes place in the context of the intimate relationship between the infant and mother. The infant's primary orientation to reality is erotic and centers on the mouth. The primary locus for significant contact with reality, therefore, is oral. The typical situation in which the infant's oral eroticism is experienced is the feeding relationship. Depending on the quality of experience with feeding contacts, the child learns to accept what is given by the warm and loving mother, to depend on that mother, and to expect that what she provides will be satisfying. The importance of the child-mother interaction here should not be underestimated. The child's basically oral orientation is largely biologically determined; the mother's feeding orientation is not only a product of biological factors but also of a complex process of personal development in which her sense of identity as a woman and as a mother plays a vital part. Any defect in her identity will thus have important consequences for the quality of the interaction between herself and her child.

The quality of the child's experience in social interaction with significant others in the environment extends to a whole complex set of interactions and experiences that are characteristic of this stage of development. The successful resolution of this initial phase of interaction entails certain orientations and dispositions that determine the subsequent course of the child's interpersonal interactions. They include a disposition to trust others, basic trust in oneself, a capacity to receive from others and to depend on them (to entrust oneself), and a sense of self-confidence. These qualities become important elements in the development of the mature personality. The unsuccessful resolution of this crisis will result in the defect of these same qualities and the relative dominance of such opposite qualities as mistrust and lack of confidence. Consequently, the designations "basic trust" and "basic mistrust" stand for a complex of personality factors characterizing the successful or unsuccessful resolution of this first crisis.

Autonomy versus Shame and Self-Doubt

The second stage of psychosexual development is that of anal eroticism. Biologically, this stage of development is marked by the formation of a fuller stool and maturation of the neuromuscular system to a point sufficient to allow control of sphincter muscles governing the retention and release of waste materials. Likewise, the anal zone becomes a source of erotic stimulation through the pleasurable sensations of retaining or releasing. On the psychosocial level, this early period is marked by the emergence in the child of a self-awareness as a separate and independent unit. Growing muscular control is accompanied by an increasing capacity for autonomous expression and self-regulation, which typically centers on problems of sphincter control of the so-called anal period. The ego thus enters into interactions of assertiveness with other wills in the social environment, particularly with the parents in the toilet-training situation. Successfully resolved, the crisis of autonomy lays the foundation of a mature capacity for self-assertion and self-expression, a capacity to respect the autonomy of others, an ability to maintain self-control without loss of self-esteem, and a capacity for rewarding and effective cooperation with others. The corresponding defect lays the foundation of the false autonomy that must feed on the autonomy of others by domination and excessive demands or of an excessive rigidity that can be identified in the fragile autonomy of the compulsive (anal) personality. The failure to achieve basic autonomy implies the lack of self-esteem that is reflected in a sense of shame and the lack of self-confidence implied in self-doubt.

Initiative versus Guilt

When the child enters the play age, the maturing organism reaches a developmental stage in which the subsystem serving the functions of locomotion and language is sufficiently organized to permit facile use. The motor equipment has reached a sufficient level of development to permit not merely the performance of motions but a wide-ranging experimentation in locomotion. The child begins to "test the limits" of this new-found capability. The child's activity becomes vigorous and intrusive. A similar crystallization of function occurs in the use of language, which becomes an exciting new toy calling for experimentation and the satisfaction of curiosity. The child's mode of activity is marked by intrusion: intrusion into other bodies by physical attack, into other people's attention by activity and aggressive talking, into space by vigorous locomotion, and into the unknown by active curiosity. All this activity is accompanied by a growing sexual curiosity and a development of the prerequisites of specifically masculine or feminine initiative, which is conditioned by the development of a phallic eroticism.

In the psychosocial sphere the child's experience is governed by an expanding imagination that must begin to mesh with the real structure, both physical and social, of the world. The child's fancy meets the nonfanciful demands of reality. Especially in regard to the area of phallic activity and sexual curiosity, the conflict takes on serious proportions. Excessive severity of rebuke or of prohibitions can bring about unnecessary repressions and can restrict the play of the child's imagination and initiative. If the crisis of initiative is successfully resolved, positive residues are provided for the development of conscience, a sense of responsibility and dependability, self-discipline, and a certain independence in the mature personality. This stage is therefore crucial for the formation of the superego, based on the introjection of authoritative, and especially parental, prohibitions. The unsuccessful resolution provides the basis for the harsh, rigid, moralistic, and self-punishing superego that serves as the dynamic source of a basic sense of guilt.

The interplay of parental prohibitions and identifications can work against the emergence of that sense of initiative that lends a certain spontaneity and freedom to the child's inquiring intrusions. The child assimilates an internalized system of parental norms and prohibitions that guide the course of behavior and provide the roots of the future development of a mature value system. If the assimilated elements are fundamentally realistic in foundation and orientation, they can be synthesized into the evolving structure of the mature ego. The pattern of identifications is well-defined and supported by mature parental identities in this instance, and parental prohibitions are balanced and reasonable. Much of the development of superego at this level is a function of parental adjustment and level of maturity. If, however, parental role functions are disturbed either in one or other degree or dimension, the child's successful resolution of this psychosocial crisis is threatened.

The child's emerging phallic interests need the support and formative influence of secure and stable identifications so that the foundations of a mature sense of sexual identity and role function can be established. The inability of the parents to provide the child with models of sexual functioning impairs the child's identification in an essential area of self-awareness. This dimension of superego formation is important for the evolution of a guilt-free sense of sexual adjustment.

Further, the assimilation of parental prohibitions and demands sets the stage for the future integration of ego and superego functioning. If parental demands are reasonable and realistic, the conjoint functioning of ego and superego is made possible. If, however, demands and prohibitions become the vehicle of parental immaturities, the superego formation is impaired by the assimilation of these immature elements, and the ground is laid for future conflict and guilt feelings. Guilt, then, arises from the disparity between the activity of the ego and the value-dependent prescriptions of the superego. Where the internalized norms of the superego are based on unresolved infantile conflicts—oedipal conflicts in Freud's terms—this primitive unreasonableness of the superego underlies guilt feelings that are unrealistic and therefore neurotic. The defect in this case is in the superego. If the value system is realistically based and oriented, guilt is still a possibility, not by reason of the inherent punitiveness of the superego, but by reason of the defection of the ego.

Industry versus Inferiority

The period of infantile (phallic) sexuality and the period of adult sexuality (puberty) are separated by the so-called latency period in which the child's interest is generally diverted to other matters. The child takes a step up from the level of imaginative exploration and play to a level in which participation in the adult world is foreshadowed. In Western culture, children are sent to school, where they begin to learn the skills that will equip them to take their places one day in adult society. Their interests turn to doing things and making things; in general, they become involved in developing the necessary technology for adult living. They are drawn away from home and its close associations and plunged into the matrix of the school system. They learn the reward systems of the school society and assimilate the values of application and diligence. They also assimilate the implicit cultural values of work and productivity. They achieve a sense of the pleasure of work, of the satisfaction of a task accomplished, and of the merit of perseverance in a difficult enterprise. In other words, normally developing children add to their evolving personality a sense of industry. The danger at this stage is that a lack of success in meeting the demands of the school society and the failure to resolve this psychosocial crisis will produce a sense of inadequacy and inferiority.

It must be remembered, of course, that the failure to achieve this sense of industry may reflect a defect in the resolution of previous crises. Excessive dependency on the emotional support of the family setting can impair the ability of the child to enter successfully into the atmosphere of competition and cooperation with peers, which is implied in the school society. In any case, the sense of inferiority can issue from the child's failure to find rewards in meeting the demands of the school setting.

Identity versus Identity Confusion

The passage to adolescent years is marked by an intense period of physiological growth and sudden maturation of genital organs. The psychosexual phase of puberty is accompanied on the psychosocial level by a kind of organization or crystallization of the residues of the preceding formative phases. The developmental preparations for participation in adult life must now begin to take a more or less definitive shape, so the adolescent must begin to establish a future role and function within adult society. The adolescent must develop a confident sense of self-awareness predicated on the ability to maintain inner sameness and continuity and on the confidence that this awareness is matched by the sameness and continuity of his or her meaning to others. This particular psychosocial crisis is therefore peculiarly vulnerable and sensitive to social and cultural influences. The context of the crisis is specifically interpersonal, and as such its successful resolution becomes all the more tenuous and problematic. In a special sense, achieving a sense of personal identity requires an awareness of the context of relations to reality within which the self forms and maintains its own proper identity.

"Who and what I am" cannot be divorced from the interaction that both links "my self" to reality and separates it from the nonego reality. Self-awareness, therefore, goes hand in hand with awareness of the other, whether that other be merely physical or personal or spiritual.

Identity implies a duality of awareness that underlies an acceptance of both poles of the experience of personal continuity. The failure of this psychosocial crisis implies a defect in awareness both of the self and of the nonego reality; it implies a failure in the recognition and acceptance of the self and the real; it implies an unclarity and a permeability of ego-boundaries that have been designated as "identity diffusion." Diffusion of identity lies at the root of many, if not most, of the adolescent problems in Western culture.

Intimacy versus Isolation

The status of adulthood is marked on the psychosexual level by the achievement of genital maturity. To Freud's mind, genital maturity meant the adequate functioning of a mature and well-adjusted personality. On the psychosocial level this development is paralleled by the establishment of significant interpersonal relationships that complement the previously formed identity in the social sphere. Typically, the emerging sexual drive focuses on another individual of the opposite sex as its object. The elements of sex identification, which are essential aspects of personal identity, are naturally expressed as established by the standards of intersex behavior of the society and culture. The intimate association of male and female in a close interpersonal union is thus an extension of their own identities, as well as a culturally approved institution (marriage). This fact does not mean that the sexual act is the only path to a sense of intimacy. From the point of view of personality development, the crucial element is the capacity to relate intimately and meaningfully with others in mutually satisfying and productive interactions. The pattern of such self-fulfilling relations will depend in large measure on the identity one has accepted as his or her own.

The failure to achieve a successful resolution of this psychosocial crisis results in a sense of personal isolation. The incapacity to establish warm and rewarding relationships with others is but a reflection of the failure to realize a secure and mature self-acceptance. Interpersonal relationships become strained, stiff, or formal. Even if a facade of personal warmth can be erected, there is a rigidly maintained inner wall that is never breached, a wall defended by intellectualization, distancing, and self-absorption.

Generativity versus Stagnation

The term "generativity" points to a primary concern with establishing the succeeding generation (through genes and genitality) and with guiding it. It must also be recognized, however, that other areas of altruistic effort cannot be excluded. Perhaps "productivity" or "creativity" would be better terms. In 1964 Erikson remarked:

> Generativity, as the instinctual power behind various forms of selfless "caring," potentially extends to whatever a man generates and leaves behind, creates and produces (or helps to produce). The ideological polarization of the Western world which has made Freud the century's theorist of sex, and Marx that of work, has, until quite recently, left a whole area of man's mind uncharted in psychoanalysis. I refer to man's *love for his works and ideas as well as for his children,* and the necessary self-verification which adult man's ego receives, and must receive, from his labor's challenge. [1964:131]

What is at stake in this phase of the emerging identity is a fuller realization of self as the expression and utilization of the fullest creative capacities within the individual. Such creativity can assume a myriad of forms, depending on the native endowment of the person; but the realized generativity is also determined to a large extent by the identity the individual has accepted and by the extent to which one is capable of interacting maturely and cooperatively with others. Consequently, the successful resolution of this depends closely on the degree of success achieved in the resolution of the two preceding phases of identity and intimacy. Moreover, true generativity has as its goal the enrichment of the lives of others; it involves a direct concern with the welfare of others, exclusive of any concern over the welfare of self. Enrichment of one's identity is a necessary by-product of generativity, but it cannot be its direct objective. It is precisely the failure to achieve a sense of generativity that promotes a certain self-absorption that expresses itself in self-indulgence, self-love, and selfishness.

Integrity versus Despair

Integrity marks the culmination of the development of the personality. It implies and depends on the successful resolution of all the preceding crises of psychosocial growth. It means the acceptance of oneself and all the aspects of life and the integration of these elements into a stable pattern of living. It implies the experience of and adjustment to the trials and troubles of life, as well as to its rewards and joys. Consequently, existence holds no fear; the ego has resigned itself to the acceptance of life itself and to the acceptance of the end of that life in death. Integrity thus represents the fully developed personality in its fullest and most mature self-realization. The failure to achieve ego-integration results often in a kind of despair and an unconscious fear of death: the one life cycle, which is given to every person as one's own, has not been accepted. The person who fails in integrity lives in basic self-contempt.

The effort toward integration that is called forth in this last fundamental crisis of the life cycle is directed by ultimate issues. It involves necessarily, as it must for the questioning and understanding animals that are humans, a confrontation with the basic issue of meaning and meaningfulness. If humankind has the innate capacity

Table 2.   Parallel Lines of Development

Instinctual Phases	Separation Individuation	Object Relations	Psychosocial Crises
Oral	Autism Symbiosis Differentiation	Primary narcissism Need-satisfying	Trust/Mistrust
Anal	Practicing Rapprochement	Need-satisfying Object constancy	Autonomy/Shame & Self-Doubt
Phallic	Object constancy Oedipal	Object constancy Ambivalence	Initiative/Guilt
Latency			Industry/Inferiority
Adolescence	Secondary in-dividuation	Object love	Identity/Identity confusion
Adulthood			Intimacy/Isolation Generativity/ Stagnation Integrity/Despair

to bring meaning into its existence, in this last crisis ultimate meaningfulness must be found or not found. Ultimate lack of meaning issues in profound despair. Ultimate meaning can either be accepted or rejected.

The parallel lines of development and their interrelation are indicated in Table 2.

SEVEN

Narcissism and the Dual Instinct Theory

THE CONCEPT of narcissism holds a pivotal position in the development of psychoanalytic theory. It was Freud's dawning realization of the importance of narcissism that led him to important modifications in his understanding of libido and his instinct theory. At the same time, Freud's examination of narcissism and its related clinical phenomena led him in the direction of an increasing concern with the origins and functions of the ego. Freud's first systematic discussion of the problem of narcissism appeared in a rather short paper published in 1914 under the title "On Narcissism." Freud's interest in the phenomenon of narcissism, however, had began as early as 1909 and persisted through the period in which he produced some of his most important theoretical writings, including his analysis of the Schreber case.

It must be said that the introduction of and focus upon narcissism have had broad implications and reverberations in psychoanalytic thinking since Freud's day. The whole problem of narcissism remains a difficult and problematic one for psychoanalysis. The problem of pathological narcissism remains a focus of active interest, thinking, and clinical concern even today. The problem has special relevance with regard to certain forms of character pathology, which are relatively resistant to therapeutic intervention.

The notions of self-love, autoeroticism, and narcissism were not newly coined by Freud. The term "narcissism" is based on the reference to the classic myth of Narcissus, who is said to have fallen in love with his own reflection in the water of a pool and to have drowned in his attempt to embrace the beloved image. The incorporation of narcissism into Freud's perspective was extremely significant in that it provided the first libidinal attachment directed toward the ego itself. This essentially violated the basic dualism of his instinct theory, which was based on the distinction between sexual-libidinal instincts and ego (self-preservative) instincts.

In 1908, Freud observed that in cases of dementia precox (schizophrenia), libido appeared to have been withdrawn from other persons and objects and turned inward. Freud concluded that this detachment of libido from external objects might account for the loss of reality contact so typical of these patients. He speculated in his 1914 discussion of narcissism that the detached libido had then been reinvested and attached to the patient's own ego. This attachment resulted in the megalomaniacal delusions of these patients, such that the libidinal investment was reflected in their grandiosity and omnipotence.

Freud also became aware at the same time that narcissism was not limited to these psychotic patients. It might also occur in neurotic and, to a certain extent, even in "normal" individuals under certain conditions. He noted, for example, that in states of physical illness and hypochondriasis, libidinal cathexis was frequently withdrawn from outside objects and from external activities and interests. Similarly, he speculated that in sleep libido was withdrawn from outside objects and reinvested in the person's own body. Thus, he thought it could be that the hallucinatory intensity of the dream experience and the intensity of the emotional quality of the dream might result from the libidinal cathexis of fantasy representations of the persons who composed the dream images. Freud also appealed to the basically narcissistic form of object choice in perversions, particularly homosexuality.

Other manifestations of narcissism were the significant role it played in the myths and beliefs of primitive people, who attributed the occurrence of external events to the magical omnipotence of their own thought processes. Particularly important is the narcissism of young children, which is relatively available even to casual observation. Children are exclusively dedicated to their own self-interest and cling tenaciously and convincedly to the magical omnipotence of their own thoughts.

Freud's observations on narcissism, particularly the behavior of very young children, provided strong evidence for the role of narcissism in development. The introduction of narcissism into his theory played a significant role because it required that he reconcile his theory of libido with what now seemed to be a libidinal force operating within the ego.

Narcissism and the Development of Object Relations

Freud postulated a state of "primary narcissism" that he said existed at birth. It is important to note that primary narcissism is a hypothetical construct that Freud postulated to integrate certain observations and theoretical formulations. For obvious reasons the hypothesis is not testable by direct observation. The postulate of primary narcissism, however, has been radically questioned in recent years, particularly under the pressure of increasing evidence that the neonate, even immediately after birth, can be quite responsive to environmental stimuli in quite complex and organized ways. Consequently, it is difficult to say whether or not such a postulated state as primary narcissism ever actually exists.

This is not to say that the neonate is not in a highly narcissistic state concerning libidinal concentration. As Freud saw it, the neonate was entirely narcissistic, one whose libidinal energies were devoted entirely to the satisfaction of physiological needs and to the preservation of a state of equilibrated well-being. The infant's basic self-investment of libido Freud termed narcissistic or "ego libido." Later on, as the infant gradually comes to recognize the principal caretaker as a source of relief of tension or pleasure, narcissistic libido is released and redirected toward investment in that person, usually the mother. Freud called this transformed libido that becomes available for attachment to external figures "object libido."

The development of object relations consequently parallels this shift from primary narcissism to object attachment—that is, from early infancy, when narcissistic libido is preeminent, to later childhood when object libido comes to dominate the libidinal organization. Note, however, that some narcissistic libido is present normally throughout adult life. From the point of view of healthy development, a healthy and well-integrated narcissism is essential for the maintenance of a sense of well-being or a sense of self-esteem in the developing personality. Like the forms of object libido, narcissistic libido can also undergo fixation and undergo developmental vicissitudes that direct it in the path of more pathological development. Freud observed that in a variety of traumatic situations (physical as well as psychological)— for example, actual injury or the threat of injury, object loss, or excessive deprivation or frustration—object libido could be withdrawn from its attachment to objects and reinvested in the ego. He called this regressive renewal of libidinal investment in the individual's own ego "secondary narcissism."

It should be noted at this juncture that Freud originally thought of the reinvestment of libido as directed to the ego as such. This formulation has given rise to a considerable confusion in the understanding of narcissistic libido. A decisive reorganization of the concept of narcissism was provided by Heinz Hartmann when he pointed out that it was more accurate to regard narcissistic libido as attached, not to the ego as such, but to the self. The proper opposition, then, between object libido and narcissistic libido is that the former is attached to objects, whereas the latter is attached to the self. This important shift in the understanding of narcissism has opened up an area of theoretical reconsideration, which is still very much in flux, and has introduced into psychoanalytic thinking the concept of self as an important, albeit as yet ill-defined, intrapsychic structural component.

The development of a concept of object relations, following Freud's original view of the transformation of narcissistic libido into object libido, has more classically been viewed in opposition to infantile narcissism. Thus, extending Freud's view, classical analysis has always viewed the development of object relations as proportional to the diminution in the titer of infantile narcissism. As children develop, their attachment to objects, at first essential for the maintenance of life, calls on a basic shift of libidinal investments from the undifferentiated and self-contained sphere of primary narcissism to the regime of object libido. As children continue to develop, the quality and nature of attachment to and involvement with objects undergo a progressive change, at each step of which the continued conversion of narcissistic libido is seen as an essential aspect of the development of object relationships.

Although this perspective was able to provide a reasonable account of the transition from pathological narcissism to various degrees of object investment and development of object relationships, it did not account very satisfactorily for the building of appropriate and adaptive degrees of narcissism into the developing psyche. Analysts would generally agree, in the contemporary context, that a healthy degree of narcissism is required for meaningful and adaptive human living and for the capacity to engage in mutually gratifying human relationships in psychologically healthy and adaptive ways. Thus, the mature love of the object in a loving relationship is sustained and supported by a degree of positive self-regard and a healthy narcissistic investment in one's own self. Clearly, in fact, the deficits of such healthy narcissism in the pathological forms of exaggerated narcissistic grandiosity or its opposite sense of inferiority or depression can have a severely detrimental effect on the individual's capacity for object relationships and on the vicissitudes of that person's particular love relationships.

Consequently, there is left a tension in points of view. On the one hand, the development of object relationships takes place only to the degree that infantile self-involvement and narcissistic self-investment can be surrendered. On the other hand, at the same time, meaningful and adult object relationships are possible only to the extent to which one can enjoy and make a significant and meaningful narcissistic investment in one's own self and in one's own self-regard. These perspectives have led to differing analytic views about narcissism: for some analysts, narcissism is always clinically detrimental and must be regarded as pathological; other analysts, however, adopting a view somewhat at variance with the classic Freudian theory, regard narcissism as undergoing a separate course of development, so that in certain degree and within certain contexts it is not only not pathological, but its own inherent development is of extreme importance for the psychological growth of the individual.

The Contribution of Heinz Kohut

This latter perspective has evolved not solely, but in large measure, from the contributions of Kohut in 1966, 1971, and 1977. In Kohut's account, the infant begins life in a state of self-contained, undifferentiated primary narcissism. His starting point, therefore, for the course of specifically narcissistic development is the same as Freud's—a primary state of undifferentiated, objectless, diffuse, and global energic containment. The first differentiation of this primitive narcissism comes in the form of two basic archaic narcissistic configurations, the "grandiose self" and the "idealized parent imago." This differentiation presumably takes place hand in hand with the emerging differentiation between self and objects that marks the passage out of the original state of primary narcissism.

Moreover, this earliest discrimination seems to take place by reason of the unavoidable conditions making it impossible for the child to maintain the primary narcissistic state, presumably contingent on that degree of frustration in maternal ministrations and responsiveness to the child's needs that brings with it the dawning realization that the child can no longer continue in the experience of being a self-contained and self-sufficient entity capable of satisfying his or her own internal needs. Rather, the existential dependence on an external object for the satisfaction of such needs and the consequent setting of limits on the child's sense of self-sufficiency and omnipotence are important developmental aspects of this process. Moreover, it should be pointed out that the earliest differentiation of archaic narcissistic states preserves an aspect of the undifferentiated narcissism as the internal possession around which the child preserves the residues of narcissistic omnipotence and grandiosity, whereas the second idealizing component relocates these residues in the external object reflected in the imago, so that the object in turn is viewed as powerful and idealized. From one point of view the child's preservation of a sense of security requires the maintenance of some residue of infantile grandiosity, whereas from another point of view the maintenance of such security requires a situation of dependence and protective symbiosis with a powerful and idealized object.

As development proceeds, each of these basic narcissistic configurations undergoes progressive modification and gradual integration in the emerging and forming psychic structure shaping the individual's internal world. This narcissistic development takes place by the continual creation and re-creation of a sequence of self-objects; that is, that the child progressively relates to objects not merely as objects existing in themselves as independent and separate entities but, rather, as modified by the addition of specific components from the child's own emerging self-organization. Such objects differ from the classically conceived objects invested with object libido because they are invested with significant degrees of narcissistic cathexis, proportional to the nature and quality of the self-derived elements that are projected onto objects in the forming of such self-objects.

The relationship with such self-objects carries on the important function of maintaining the internal narcissistic equilibrium, which requires continual readjustment in the face of the sequence of narcissistic vulnerabilities arising at various phases of the developmental process. Thus, at the earliest infantile phase of such development, the child might relate to the mother as a self-object in a quite symbiotic way: mother and child are merged as a psychic unit that allows only the faintest hint of distancing between mother and child as separate foci of psychic activity. The child's sense of continuing availability and lack of separateness between child and mother serves a stabilizing function for the child's need to preserve an inner sense of narcissistic balance. In such a context, premature separation between the child and the essential self-object would throw the child's fragile sense of self into a severe state of deprivation and fragmentation, the implications of which would be equivalent to psychic annihilation.

As development proceeds, however, the child's dependence on the mother and the quality of the self-object relationship shift so that the vulnerability is concerned less with loss of the mother and more with loss of the mother's love. The connection with the mother, however, remains essential for the maintenance of the child's narcissistic equilibrium and coherence. At some point in development, the child reaches a state where such internal cohesiveness and the integrity of evolving psychic structures allow a preservation of a sense of inner continuity and cohesiveness of self-organization not only when realizing the potential loss of the object, or even the loss of love of the object, but when met by other narcissistic disappointments and vulnerabilities as well. The establishment of such inner narcissistic cohesion in the self-organization is an important developmental acquisition; it distinguishes between those conditions in which the individual is capable of maintaining the integrity of narcissistic structures when facing external threats and those forms of pathology in which regression and fragmentation of narcissistic structures take place in the face of narcissistic losses or traumata.

At each stage in this developmental progression, the original archaic narcissistic formations, the grandiose self and the idealized parent imago, undergo progressive modifications, so that at each phase of the progression the degree of narcissistic investment is modified in more modulated and realistic directions, and thus at each stage there is a proportional transformation of these narcissistic structures into more constructive, stable, and autonomous psychic structures. Consequently, the grandiose self is gradually modified in more realistic directions that allow the child to maintain a sense of self-esteem and pride in accomplishment, even when confronted with unavoidable disappointments and with the acknowledgment of given limitations. Ultimately, the grandiose self is modified in the direction of a mature sense of stable and secure self-esteem, pride in accomplishment, ambition, and the resilient capacity to maintain narcissistic balance despite severe losses and narcissistic disappointments. Similarly, the idealized parental imago is modified progressively in the direction of a realistic and attainable ego ideal that is gradually internalized as a meaningful and sustaining set of personal values and ideals.

At any stage of this process, the reworking of the elements of archaic narcissism can be interfered with and undergo a variety of pathological vicissitudes. The results of such developmental impediments will be a variety of forms of narcissistic disorder, stretching from severe narcissistic vulnerability and the threat of disillusion and fragmentation of the self to higher orders of narcissistic vulnerability in which the threat of loss of self-cohesion is minimal, but in which various forms of pathological behavior can emerge as a result of narcissistic disappointment, threat, or trauma. Ultimately, the transformation of narcissism finds its most mature and realistic expression in the capacity for creativity, for empathy, for humor, for wisdom and, finally, for the acceptance of transience and the inevitability of death.

Narcissism versus Autoeroticism

An important question raised by the consideration of narcissism is its difference from and relation to autoeroticism. In fact, the difference between the two is fundamental. For primary narcissism, there is no differentiation of self and object and no quality of object-involvement in the infant's libidinal experience. Autoeroticism refers to eroticism in relationship to the subject's own body or its parts. If the child cannot have the love object (mother) or the part-object (breast) desired, gratification may be sought by use of the child's own body parts (thumb sucking, for example) as if they were objects. Any erogenous zone may be used for this purpose. The capacity to gratify sexual needs in this way is autoeroticism. Autoeroticism, moreover, implies an absence of any specific object involvement. Secondary narcissism differs in that it refers specifically to the self, rather than to the subject's body or its parts. Thus, there is considerable overlap between autoeroticism and primary narcissism, although they emphasize different aspects of the primitive libidinal condition. Autoeroticism, however, is quite distinct and different from secondary narcissism.

It must be concluded, then, that the vicissitudes of narcissism are mingled with and operating throughout the entire course of psychosexual development. Waelder (1960) has made an initial attempt to apply the levels of self-love or narcissism to the developmental schemata of erotogenic zones within the framework of Freud's theory of infantile sexuality. Thus, in the oral period, narcissism is expressed as a wish for affection, a wish to be given to, and is defined as receptive narcissism. The narcissism of the phallic period designates a wish for admiration, which is said to characterize the phallic stage of psychosexual development.

Moreover, at each stage of psychosexual development the child is open to narcissistic insult of a kind that is phase-specific and related both to the vicissitudes of object libido and the state of internal development of the psychic apparatus. Thus, oral deprivation can also be envisioned as narcissistic injury, contributing to the undermining of the infant's sense of inner value or worth. Similarly, the vicissitudes of the oedipal period have a strong narcissistic component, which opens the child to narcissistic mortification by reason of the disappointment of oedipal wishes that can leave a sense of inadequacy, inferiority, or lack of value. Narcissistic injury at these various points of the developmental program can leave the child with an emerging sense of shame and self-embarrassment and with a variety of other vulnerabilities that can be the nidus of later forms of character pathology or other psychopathology.

Narcissism and the Choice of Love Object

Reference was made earlier to the crucial role of early object relationships in the later choice of love objects. Freud had found that a deepened understanding of the vicissitudes of narcissism made it easier to understand the basis for choice of certain love objects in adult life. A love object might be chosen, as Freud put it, "according to the narcissistic type," that is, because the object resembles the subject's idealized self-image (or fantasied self-image). Possibly the choice of object might be an "anaclitic type," in which case the object might resemble someone who took care of the subject during the early years of life. Freud felt that certain personalities that have a high degree of narcissism, especially certain types of beautiful women, have an appeal over and above their aesthetic attraction. Such women supply for their lovers the lost narcissism that was painfully renounced in the process of turning toward a love object. Another important category in which the narcissistic type of object choice plays a significant role is that of homosexuality. In the homosexual object relationship, the individual's choice of the object is predicated on the resemblance of the object to the subject's own body, with its similarity of sexual organs.

In summary, the concept of narcissism occupies a central and pivotal position in psychoanalytic theory. With the introduction of the concept of narcissism, it became obvious that the concept of the "individual" and the individual's "body" and "ego" could no longer be used interchangeably. It became clear that further understanding and advances in psychoanalytic theory would depend on a clearer definition of the concept of self and its more adequate delineation from the concept of ego. Attempts to implement such understanding have brought into focus the ambiguities in the concept of the ego and have underscored the need for the systematic study of its development, structure, and functions. Attention to narcissistic phenomena has also enlarged the understanding of a variety of mental disorders, as well as various normal psychological phenomena. These issues will be discussed in chapter 11.

Aggression and Ego Instincts

The aggressive drives hold a peculiar place in Freud's theory. His thinking about aggression underwent a gradual evolution. Early in his thinking, his attention had been preoccupied by the problems posed by libidinal drives. He was quite aware of the aggressive components often expressed in the operation of libidinal factors, but he could not long avoid taking explicit account of the more destructive aspects of instinctual functioning. Undoubtedly, also, the horrors and destructiveness of World War I made a significant impression on him, so that he began to realize more profoundly the significance of destructive urges in human behavior.

By 1915, in his "Instincts and Their Vicissitudes," Freud had arrived at a dualistic conception of the instincts as divided into sexual instincts and ego instincts. He recognized a sadistic component of the sexual instincts, but this still lacked a sound theoretical basis. Oral, anal, and phallic levels of development all had their sadistic components. Devoid of any manifest eroticism, and covering a wide range from sexual perversions to impulses of cruelty and destructiveness, the sadistic aspects certainly had different aims from the more strictly libidinal.

Increasingly, Freud saw the sadistic component as independent of the libidinal and gradually segregated it from the libidinal drives. Moreover, impulses to control, tendencies toward the acquisition and exercise of power, and defensive trends toward attacking and destroying, all manifested a strong element of aggressiveness. It seemed, then, that there was sadism associated with the ego instincts, as well as with the libidinal instincts. Freud once again followed the dualistic bent of his mind and postulated two groups of instinctual impulses, two qualitatively different and independent sources of instinctual impulses with different aims and modalities.

The problem, of course, was that in certain areas these two instincts seemed to work in conjunction, whereas in other areas they seemed to be in opposition. Thus, the notion of "sadism" was gradually broadened to include other characteristics under the heading of aggressiveness. At this point in his thinking Freud attributed aggressiveness to the ego instincts and thus separated the sadistic components from the sexual instincts and preserved the duality. This view also asserted the independent character of the ego instincts. Sexual sadism was then explained by the fusion between ego instincts and sexual instincts. This fusion was the converse of the admixture of libidinal impulses with the ego instincts in narcissism. However, there were two problems in this rearrangement of the instinct theory. First, the criterion for distinguishing instincts had shifted from the source of the instinct to its aim. Second, the basic concept of instinct that comprehended it as a mechanism for discharge for energic tension, although still at least theoretically applicable to the sexual instincts, was difficult to apply to the ego instincts.

Putting the aggressive instinct in the category of ego instincts, however, had its further difficulties. The classification gave rise to still another problem. On the basis of clinical evidence of the self-destructive tendencies of depressed patients and the self-inflicted injury among masochistic patients, along with his observations of the wanton destructiveness normally manifested by small children, Freud concluded that in many instances aggression or aggressive impulses did not serve self-preservative purposes. Therefore, it seemed contradictory that they should be assigned to the ego instincts. The difficulties made it necessary for Freud to take an additional step. The next step involved removing aggressiveness from the ego instincts and separating it out from the ego.

With the publication of *The Ego and the Id* in 1923, Freud gave aggression a separate status as an instinct with a separate source, which he postulated to be largely the skeletomuscular system, and a separate aim of its own, namely, destruction. Aggression was no longer a component instinct, nor was it a characteristic of the ego instincts; it was an independently functioning instinctual system with aims of its own.

The elevation of aggression to the status of a separate instinct, on a par with sexual instincts, dealt a severe blow to any lingering romantic notions of the essentially or exclusively good nature of man. Aggression and destructiveness were seen as inherent qualities of human nature, such that aggressive impulses were elicited when an individual was sufficiently thwarted or abused. Freud's new formulation also drew attention to the specific role of aggression in forms of psychopathology, as well as attention to the understanding of the developmental processes through which aggression could be normally integrated and controlled.

The progressive development of aggression is an important component of both the developing infant's capacity to engage with, control, and manipulate the environment and the infant's increasing engagement in meaningful relationships with objects. The early precursors of aggression are manifested in forms of crying and distress and are primarily a vehicle of essential communication that serves to elicit appropriate responses from objects. The high point of the infant's specific libidinal attachment to the mother at about five months is followed by increasing efforts to differentiate from and detach from the mother in the interest of exploring the world. The mother's efforts to restrain this exuberant and often dangerous exploration are met by anger and struggle against the mother's restraints. This anger toward and attacks against the mother emerge at about eight to ten months, whereas previously attacks against the object with intent to hurt cannot be observed. This capacity for directing anger against the mother is a function of the infant's more stable libidinal cathexis of the mother and development of the capacity to experience anger in a more organized fashion. Moreover, the anger occurs in connection with unpleasureful restriction or frustration of activity, and as soon as the obstruction is removed, the anger subsides. Anger at this level is stimulus-bound, short-lived, and restricted to specific eliciting conditions.

Gradually, defensive modifications of aggression become observable, particularly through the displacement, restriction of aim, sublimation, and fusion with libido of aggressive impulses. The infant becomes playfully teasing or begins to displace anger at the mother toward a doll or, even, turns it inward. Patterns of inhibition, withdrawal, or negativism begin to be seen. The rapid alternation between loving affection and angry attacks has been described as "ambitendency." By twelve months of age, the infant's object-directed anger has become more differentiated, integrated, and complex, without as yet manifesting any deliberate intent to hurt. Under optimal conditions anger can be used constructively in the service of distancing and promoting self-object differentiation. When conditions are unfavorable, as in the case of overly controlling, intrusive, or anxious mothers, the infant's excessive anger, frequently accompanied with anxiety, tends to interfere with optimal distancing. Such infants will often show patterns of excessive avoidance or excessive clinging to the mother.

Such patterns undoubtedly reflect the premature differentiation of aggression related to a failure of need-satisfying responses from the object. The consequence is an increased cathexis of the object with aggression, an increased titer of ambivalence, and a perception of the object as frustrating and bad. The difficulties posed by an excessive titer of aggression and ambivalence for the accomplishing of distancing behaviors in the practicing subphase also contribute to difficulties in self-object differentiation. It is not until the young child enters the rapprochement subphase with its more differentiated and stable representations of both self and object that aggression can be expressed in any more sustained fashion and begins to approximate forms of aggression at more adult levels, including the intent to hurt.

It should be noted that aggression remains a problem for psychoanalytic thinking even today. Although a great deal has been learned about the operation and vicissitudes of aggression since Freud originally struggled with it, there is still a great deal that remains to be learned about its nature, its origins, the conditions that produce and unleash it, as well as the developmental factors that contribute to its pathological deviations and to its more constructive integration in the realm of human functioning.

Pleasure Principle and Reality Principle

From the very beginning of Freud's thinking, he envisioned the instincts as governed by certain regulatory principles that were applied to all stimuli impinging on the organism—both stimuli emanating from the external environment and stimuli emanating from within the organism (Table 1). Even at the time of the writing of the *Project* in 1895, Freud recognized the importance of the constancy principle, that is, a tendency of the organism to maintain a particular state or level of energic equilibrium. Further, the Nirvana principle was a logical extension of the notions of entropy and constancy, which postulated a tendency on the part of the organism to discharge any internal tension in an effort to lower the levels of internal tension in the direction of seeking a state of complete cessation of stimuli or release of tension.

The pleasure principle, thus, was largely an application of these more fundamental regulatory principles. Freud viewed the pleasure principle as an inborn tendency of the organism to avoid pain and seek pleasure, through the release of tension by way of energic discharge. The immediate discharge of tension, however, is not always possible. Inevitably, then, the demands of the pleasure principle must be modified. The demands of reality necessitate the capacity for delay of pleasure—that is, postponement of immediate release of tension—

with the aim of achieving even greater pleasure in the long run. Thus, the reality principle modifies the pleasure principle to meet the demands of external reality. The reality principle arises out of the organism's continual experience of the frustration imposed by the conditions of reality and thus is largely a learned function. Consequently, it is closely related to maturation of ego functions and may be impaired in a variety of mental disorders resulting from impeded ego development. Here again is one of the theoretical propositions in Freud's "middle period" that underscores in a particularly striking way the deficiencies of an isolated instinct theory and the need for the operation of a systematic psychology of ego and its functions.

Life and Death Instincts

When Freud introduced his final theory of life and death instincts in *Beyond the Pleasure Principle* in 1920, he took what can now be seen as an inevitable and logical next step in the evolution of the instinct theory he had been developing. It was nonetheless a highly speculative attempt to extrapolate the directions in which his instinct theory was taking shape to the broad realm of biological principles. One can recall that Freud's thinking about the instincts always cast its shadow in a dual modality. In the beginning he had distinguished sexual and ego instincts. This distinction provided the basic dichotomy for the explanation of psychological conflict and the understanding of psychoneurosis.

The concept of narcissism, however, created a breach in the independent existence of the ego instincts and revealed the operation of libidinal instincts within the ego. Consequently, the dualistic character of the instinct theory was undermined in favor of a monistic view of instincts as entirely libidinal. Moreover, the distinction of instincts with reference to their source was replaced by reclassification of instincts according to their relations to objects. Freud tried to save the ego instincts by referring to the idea of "ego interests," which he took to mean a form of nonlibidinal investment in the ego. The vacancy in the ego instincts, which resulted from the inroads of narcissism, was filled to a certain extent by the gradual separation of the aggressive instinct as a separate entity, which Freud could then locate in the ego and identify with ego instincts. The inconsistency, however, between the concept of aggressiveness and sadism, along with the alternate fusion and opposition between sadistic and libidinal impulses, led Freud to the next step of separating both libidinal and aggressive instincts from the ego and locating them in the vital stratum of the mind, the id, which was quite independent of the ego. Thus, the ego was left with its own "ego instincts," the nature of which at that point remained unspecified.

The introduction of the life and death instincts must be seen in the course of this development and as extending the inherent duality of instinctual theory to the level of ultimate and final biological principle. Freud had not divorced his notion from the underlying economic principles, which were derived from the principle of entropy and constancy. The constancy principle was extended to the Nirvana principle, which objective was cessation of all stimuli or a state of total rest. It was only a small, subsequent step that led Freud from the formulation of a Nirvana principle to the death instinct, or *Thanatos*. Freud thus postulated that the death instinct was a tendency of all organisms and their component cells to return to a state of total quiescence; that is, to an inanimate state.

In opposition to this instinct he set the life instinct, or *Eros*, which referred to the tendencies for organic particles to reunite, of parts to bind to one another to form greater unities, as in sexual reproduction. As Freud viewed the matter, the ultimate destiny of all biological matter, driven by the inexorable tendencies of all life to follow the principles of entropy and constancy (with the exception of the germ plasm), was to return to an inanimate state. He felt that the dominant force in biological organisms had to be the death instinct. In this final formulation of life and death instincts, the instincts were considered to represent abstract biological principles, which transcended the operation of libidinal and aggressive drives. The life and death instincts represented the forces that underlie the sexual and aggressive instincts. Consequently, they represented a general trend in all biological organisms.

In evaluating these general biological, instinctual principles, one must realize that Freud was engaging in a somewhat exorbitant speculation. He in no way believed that the death instinct, for example, was clinically verifiable. He did think that certain clinical phenomena suggested that a more general principle, such as the death instinct, may be operating, but he in no way thought that the observations could be used to demonstrate such principles. He pointed in particular to the tendency of persons to repeat past patterns of behavior (repetition compulsion), even when such behavior has proved to be ill-advised or self-defeating. He also pointed to the evidence of strong masochistic needs in many neurotic patients.

Needless to say, Freud's extravagant speculation has been subjected to severe criticism. It is impossible to argue from the basis of clinical observation to such a general biological principle as a conclusion. If the inherent destructiveness of some states of psychopathology can permit the inference of destructive forces operating in the individual psyche, it by no means points to the existence of inherent and biologically determined forces of self-destructive potential. However one regards the argument as a biological speculation, it has little relevance as a psychological speculation. Consequently, the vast majority of contemporary psychoanalysts, although they strongly endorse Freud's dual instinct theory, either reject or pass over in silence the further extension of his theory to life and death.

One significant group of psychoanalytic theorists is a marked exception to this view. The school of analysts who have followed the lead of Melanie Klein bases a considerable portion of its understanding of intrapsychic processes on the operation of the life and death instincts. In Klein's work with severely disturbed children, she ascribed the manifestations of aggressive instincts in such children to the operation of the death instinct. This point of view seems to collapse the intervening steps in the organization of instinctual theory and makes almost any manifestation of destructive aggression a direct expression of the death instinct. Although the contributions of Klein and her followers to the psychopathology of childhood disturbances are significant, other schools of analytic thinking have not followed their lead in this conceptualization of the primary instincts.

Moreover, the implicit parallelism in the organization and economy of separate instincts—libidinal and aggressive—that was embedded in Freud's systematic thinking about these instincts is currently under severe questioning and has been subjected to vigorous criticism. It is not at all apparent that the operation of aggressive instincts can be conceived of in terms analogous to that of libido. Consequently, the whole understanding of the relationship between these separate instinctual drives, their relative economy, their relationship and integration with the structures and functions of both ego and superego are currently undergoing considerable rethinking.

EIGHT

Nature and Origins
of Anxiety

ONE OF THE most significant parameters in the development of Freud's thinking came in relation to the theory of anxiety. The initial theory and its evolution and replacement by a subsequent formulation parallel the current of development that was taking place in other aspects of Freud's thought, most notably his instinct theory. Particularly significant in relation to the theory of anxiety was the shift from a primarily physiological-energic-organismic basis to a formulation that was specifically psychological. Accompanying this progression in his thinking was the repositioning of anxiety from instinctual foundations to ego functions.

Initial Formulations

Freud's initial theory of anxiety placed the emphasis on its biological genesis in the sexual instinct. As a result of his early clinical study in the 1890s, pathological anxiety was uniformly and univocally attributed to disturbances in sexual functioning. His theorizing focused on the etiology of anxiety in specific clinical entities. He distinguished two important groups of pathology in which anxiety played a major role. First, he classified a group of syndromes that he denominated as the "actual neuroses." This group included neurasthenia, hypochondriasis, and anxiety neurosis. *Neurasthenia* was a state of chronic impoverishment and fatigue in which patients were generally apathetic, disinterested, moody, suffering from a paralyzing fatigue caused by an impoverishment of energy and a tension and restlessness caused by warded-off impulses demanding discharge. These patients feel the necessity for an outlet but, nevertheless, lack enthusiasm and interest in any outlet that might be offered. *Hypochondriasis* was a form of organ neurosis manifesting itself in stressful and painful bodily sensations. *Anxiety neurosis* was a state of restless agitation and perturbation in which the patient suffered from apparently unmotivated emotional attacks, chiefly anxiety spells, along with disturbances of physical function that were partly inhibition and partly anxiety equivalents. In all of the actual neuroses, Freud felt that the causative factors had a physical basis. Second, he contrasted these anxiety states to the psychoneuroses, such as hysteria or obsessive-compulsive neurosis, in which the basis of the symptoms was primarily due to psychological factors.

According to Freud, an increase in sexual tension as a purely physiological phenomenon leads to an increase in the mental representation of the sexual instinct, together with a variety of associated ideas and emotions. In the normal course of events, increased sexual tension seeks discharge somatically through sexual intercourse. Concurrently, there is a discharge of mental energy. However, in the actual neuroses, such as anxiety neurosis, abnormal sexual practices, including coitus interruptus and masturbation, prevent the proper somatic discharge of sexual tensions or "toxins." Concomitantly, the adequate expression of the psychic elaboration of these sexual tensions is also inhibited or distorted. Freud maintained that it was this interference with the adequate discharge of the psychic component of sexual tension—that is, its specifically libidinal aspects—that gives rise to anxiety. Freud contrasted this situation to the etiology of anxiety in psychoneurotic states, such as hysteria or obsessive-compulsive neurosis, which were due to psychological causes, specifically the interference with normal libidinal functioning caused by psychic conflict or repression. The symptoms of the actual neurosis—anxiety accompanied by weakness, fatigue, rapid or irregular heart action, constipation, excessive sweating, and other vague somatic complaints—were often indistinguishable from those of psychoneurosis. They could only be adequately distinguished in the light of the patient's history and the total clinical picture.

It is clear at this point that Freud held a dual theory of the etiology of anxiety or, more accurately, two separate theories. The one theory was a theory of toxic (physiological) origin, in which the anxiety was the result of dammed-up and undischarged libido that was thereby forced to seek abnormal physiological discharge in the anxiety symptom. The second theory was also related to the patient's sexual malfunction, but the etiology lay at a more specifically psychological level; namely, in the repression of libidinal urges typically thought of as derived from unconscious infantile memories.

Although it is particularly striking that Freud should have maintained a toxic view of anxiety, his strong physicalistic bias and the powerful urge that he felt to root his study of the functioning of the mind, and the pathological disturbances related to it, in bodily functioning are known.

The actual neuroses were an important area in which Freud felt that he had identified a specific etiology that explained the nature and origin of the anxiety symptoms. Freud maintained his view of the toxic etiology of anxiety, as at least one area of somatically based anxiety, nearly to the end of his career. The basic notion of anxiety as transformed libido continued to be a part of his thinking. At the same time, however, there were subtle shifts in the concept of libido itself. It had begun its career as a largely physiological concept but gradually shifted more and more so that it became something of a border concept between the physiological and psychological realms. It was not really until 1933, in the *New Introductory Lectures,* that the hypothesis of anxiety as transformed libido was finally rejected altogether, even though Freud had radically revised and extended his theory of anxiety and had completely shifted and reoriented his thinking about instincts.

Difficulties with the Early Theory

It should be noted, first of all, that psychoanalytic investigators have differed rather broadly in their views about Freud's formulations on the actual neuroses. There are investigators who have considered the actual neuroses as valid and meaningful concepts, just as there are those who have not only questioned the validity of Freud's toxic theory of anxiety but even the validity of the clinical entities themselves. For a long time, one of the main objections to Freud's toxic theory was on the basis of his postulating sexual substances related to the toxic aspects of sexual functioning. In the intervening years, however, endocrinological research has confirmed the existence of a surprising variety of sexual "substances," the sex hormones. Freud's speculations were not so absurd, although imbalances of sexual hormones may have little to do with anxiety as a psychological phenomenon. The roles of norepinephrine and other hormonal and neurotransmitter substances in the elaboration of anxiety are yet to be determined.

Nonetheless, Freud's early theory of anxiety had certain inherent limitations. First, it contradicted a basic aspect of the psychoanalytic concept of the psychoneurosis: Freud had postulated that in the psychoneurosis anxiety was the result of sexual repression. If repression is the agency for the production of anxiety, repression must therefore precede anxiety. What then was the cause of repression? Freud had also observed that repression arose in response to unbearable affects, which would certainly include anxiety. Moreover, in certain clinical cases it was found that with the lifting or loosening of repression, instead of the patients getting better, they became even more severely anxiety ridden and panicked. This unfortunate clinical outcome could not have been expected if repression were simply the cause of anxiety. The obvious alternative was, of course, that anxiety somehow preceded, and was causally related to, repression. The conflict between these two alternatives represented a source of considerable uncertainty and controversy in early analytic circles.

Second, the theory did not take into account anxiety that arises in response to realistic danger; that is, the so-called objective anxiety. In certain situations, the anticipation of external danger may cause somatic responses and subjective sensations of fear, which are indistinguishable from those that occur in neurotic states. These conditions, however, are entirely unrelated to the accumulation of sexual tension or of toxic sexual substances.

In struggling with these difficulties in his theory, Freud came to realize that anxiety can best be understood, not through its associated sensations or somatic expression, but rather by whether it is precipitated by an external or internal danger. In other words, a comprehensive theory of anxiety must take into account its relationship to the self-preservative goals of the organism. The deficiencies involved in Freud's early theory of anxiety underscored the inevitable limitations of an approach that tries to account for a phenomenon as complex as anxiety entirely on the basis of consideration of the instincts and their vicissitudes, without reference to the functions of other levels and aspects of the psychic apparatus or its relationship to the outside world.

Freud's initial theory was rooted in his early thinking about instinctual processes, specifically the sexual etiology of psychopathology. The basically toxic and physiological rudiments of this theory reveal to a surprising degree the extent to which Freud's physicalistic bias influenced the entire tenor of his thinking. Even the emendations and extensions of his later theories of anxiety did not discard the important relationship between frustrated sexuality and anxiety in certain neurotic conditions; nor did it rule out the possibility that there was a direct somatic relationship between sexual conflict and anxiety, the precise nature of which had not as yet been defined. In the modified theory, however, he was able to incorporate these economic considerations within a broader and more meaningful theoretical framework.

The new theory of anxiety was enunciated in Freud's *Inhibitions, Symptoms, and Anxiety*, which appeared in 1926. The date is important because it means that the revision of the anxiety theory came a few years after the 1923 publication of *The Ego and the Id*, in which Freud had presented the important theoretical reorientation by which he abandoned the topographic model and put in its place the structural model. Consequently, the revision in the theory of anxiety was prepared for by the gradual emergence of Freud's structural views and his increasing awareness of the importance and functioning of the ego. In contrast to the earlier theory, which approached anxiety from the standpoint of the drives, the new theory attacked the problem from the standpoint of the ego. It set aside the biological approach to anxiety. The physiological aspect of anxiety remained a subject of research chiefly in disciplines outside of psychoanalysis proper.

The new theory focused on the function of anxiety in relation to a variety of threats to the organism, both from within and from without. Both "real" anxiety and neurotic anxiety were now viewed as occurring in response to a danger to the organism. In real anxiety the threat emanated from a known danger outside of the individual. In neurotic anxiety the danger was precipitated from an unknown source, a source that was not necessarily external.

Anxiety as a Signal of Danger

Freud distinguished in his new theory two kinds of anxiety-provoking situations. In the first, which took as its prototype the phenomenon of birth, anxiety occurred as a result of excessive instinctual stimulation that the organism does not have the capacity to bind or handle. In this type of situation, which arises because of the helpless state of the individual, the excessive accumulation of instinctual energy overruns the protective barriers of the ego and a state of panic or trauma results. These traumatic states are most likely to occur in infancy or childhood, when the ego is relatively immature. They may also occur in adult life, however, particularly in states of psychotic turmoil or panic states, when the ego organization is overwhelmed by the threatening danger.

The more common situation, which occurs typically after the defensive organization of the psyche has matured, is that anxiety arises in anticipation of danger, rather than as its result. The anxiety that is subjectively experienced may be evoked by a circumstance that is similar to a danger that had already occurred. In these situations the affect of anxiety serves a protective function by signaling to the subject the approach of danger. The signal of danger may arise because the individual has learned to recognize, at a preconscious or unconscious level, aspects of a situation that had once proven to be traumatic. Thus, the anxiety serves as a signal for the ego to mobilize protective measures, which can then be directed toward averting the danger and preventing a traumatic situation from arising. The dangers may arise from external sources, but they may also arise from internal sources; namely, the threatening of the ego or the potential overwhelming of its defenses by instinctual drives. The individual may use avoidance mechanisms to escape from a real or imagined danger from without, or the ego may bring to bear psychological defenses within itself to guard against or reduce the quantity of instinctual excitation. As Anna Freud has pointed out, to a certain extent the defensive mechanisms of the ego may also function to avoid external dangers, as well as internal ones.

According to this revised theory of anxiety, such neurotic symptoms as phobias indicate a partial defect in the psychic apparatus. Specifically, in phobias the defensive activity of the ego has not succeeded in adequately coping with the threatening drive manifestations. Consequently, mental conflict persists, and the danger that actually arose from within is now externalized and treated as if it had its origins in the external world, at least in part. Thus, neurosis can be regarded as a failure in the defensive function of the ego, and this failure results in a distortion of the ego's relationship to some aspect of the outside world. In psychotic states the failure of defensive function is more complete, and the potential threat to the fragile ego and its permeable defenses is all the more overwhelming and annihilating. Thus, greater portions of external reality are perceived as overwhelmingly threatening, and greater distortions of the ego become necessary to accommodate the distortions in the patient's view of the outside world.

Characteristic Danger Situations

Each stage of the child's development is accompanied by characteristic danger situations that are phase-specific or "appropriate" to the issues pertinent to that particular developmental phase. Thus, the earliest danger situation, which occurs when the child is most immature and psychologically and physiologically vulnerable and helpless, is the loss of the primary object; that is, the caretaking and nurturing person on whom the child is entirely dependent. Later, when the value of the object itself begins to be perceived, the fear of losing the object's love then exceeds the fear of losing the object itself. The whole developmental effort of the child to separate physically and psychologically from dependence on the primary symbiotic objects and the necessary developmental steps toward increasing individuation are all subject to the concomitant threats of loss of the object or loss of the object's love.

In the phallic phase of development, however, the fear of bodily injury or castration assumes a prominent influence. This fear may be thought of as a variety of fear of loss; in this instance, though, the loss is that of a narcissistically treasured part of the body. Further on in the latency period, the characteristic fear is that parental representatives, in the internalized form of the superego, will be angry with, punish, or cease to love the child. Consequently, in each of these phases, anxiety arises in the ego. Freud also noted that although each of these determinants of anxiety was phase-related and functioned in reference to a particular developmental period, they could exist side by side in the contemporaneous ego. Furthermore, the individual's anxiety reaction to a particular danger situation might occur after the emergence from the developmental phase with which that situation was associated. The persistence in later years of anxiety reactions, which were appropriate to various pregenital phases of development, has important implications for the understanding of psychopathology. The persistence of such earlier forms of anxiety in later stages of development is a reflection of neurotic fixations at earlier stages of development, as well as a persistence of the characteristic conflicts of such earlier stages.

Implications of the New Theory of Anxiety

The first significant point relative to Freud's revision of his theory of anxiety is that it marks a decisive shift in emphasis away from a basically physiological perspective on anxiety to a perspective that is more decisively psychological. The theory of signal anxiety thus marks itself off from the earlier theory of toxic, dammed-up libido as the source of anxiety. Although Freud still clung to his toxic theory, the new theory introduced a more meaningful concept of anxiety, as related to anticipation of danger, so that it has much broader application and much greater explanatory power.

The second important implication of the new theory was that it marked a decisive shift in the direction of Freud's thinking about the ego. As will be discussed in chapter 9, when Freud introduced his structural theory in 1923, although he defined the ego as an important regulatory agency in the psychic economy, it was a relatively weak and fragile ego that could only survive by more or less passively responding to the powerful drives of the id and the stringent demands of the superego. The introduction of the signal theory of anxiety changed that picture of the ego in important if subtle ways. The new theory, which placed anxiety before the exercise of repression, signified that the ego enjoyed a certain amount of control over the powerful instinctual forces of the id and that it enjoyed a certain degree of autonomy in the exercise of certain of its important functions. By implication, then, the ego had resources of its own that it could bring to bear in the management and direction of unconscious impulses and in the institution of defense against the threatening upsurge of instinctual drives. The implications of this shift in the conceptualization of the ego and its functions will be spelled out more in detail in the consideration of the structural theory.

The new theory of anxiety, then, was of great potential value in clarifying the understanding of a variety of psychological phenomena. At the same time, several fundamental questions remain unanswered. It is necessary to further understand the conditions or circumstances under which the ego becomes overwhelmed by anxiety, beyond its precipitation by the anticipation of danger. Similarly, little is known about the normal psychology of anxiety. More knowledge is needed about the quantitative and qualitative factors that determine whether a given amount of anxiety will spur ego development through the mobilization and stimulation of the individual's ego potential or whether the same quantity of anxiety will impede ego development by drawing the existing ego defenses into excessive conflict formations.

A subsequent implication of the signal theory of anxiety that has only begun to be explored by analytic theorists is the idea that anxiety is an important stimulus to structural growth and that an important index of intrapsychic development and integration is the increasing capacity to tolerate anxiety. The basic idea is that the ego must somehow learn to develop the capacity to use increasing degrees of anxiety to elicit its own inner resources for mastering anxiety and thus enlarging its capacity for internal mastery and control. By implication, the factors contributing to psychic growth that would minimize or eliminate or alleviate anxiety could only undermine the important aspects of psychic development that contribute ultimately in a healthy ego to ego resourcefulness and strength. Obviously, this aspect of the theory of signal anxiety has profound implications for the treatment process, particularly in regard to its concerns for stimulating the inner growth and development of the patient.

It was also in relation to the signal theory of anxiety that Freud once again returned with renewed interest to the concept of defense. In his earlier dealings with psychic conflict in relation to the topographic model, Freud had minimized the notion of defense, reducing it somewhat simplistically to the notion of repression. It was his insight into the nature of anxiety as a signal function that brought him back to a formulation of defense mechanisms as such. He began to see that the anxiety signal stimulated mobilization of a variety of forms of defense. He began to see that repression was only one, although a very important, form of defense mechanism that the ego could employ. The variety of defenses he now saw also included reaction formation, isolation, and undoing. With the development of the signal theory of anxiety, the ego was no longer a passive agency, helpless and vulnerable in the face of the demands of the id and the outside world. It was now credited not only as a kind of advance guard, which could signal danger ahead of time, but also as having at its disposal a variety of possible responses to danger from without or within, responses that would enable it to meet the demands and threats either from the drives or from the outside world. The ego had thus become a more forceful character on the stage of the intrapsychic drama, and the way was prepared for the subsequent elaboration of its autonomous function and capacities.

NINE

Structural Theory and Ego Psychology

THE TOPOGRAPHIC theory was essentially a transitional model in the development of Freud's thinking. It served an important function in providing a framework for the development of his basic instinct theory, which, as discussed previously, was undergoing considerable revision and rethinking during that quarter century. However, the topographic theory underscores, once again, the need for a more systematic concept of psychic structure.

The main deficiency of the topographic model lies in its inability to account for two extremely important characteristics of mental conflict. Freud only became aware of these aspects of mental life by dint of a long accumulation of clinical experience with his psychoanalytic patients. The first important problem was that Freud found that many of the defense mechanisms that his patients used to avoid pain or unpleasure, and which appeared in the form of unconscious resistance during the psychoanalytic treatment, were themselves not initially accessible to consciousness. He drew the obvious conclusion that the agency of repression, therefore, could not be identical with the preconscious, because this region of the mind was by definition easily accessible to consciousness. The second problem was that he found that his patients frequently exhibited an unconscious need for punishment or an unconscious sense of guilt. According to the topographic model, however, the moral agency making this demand was allied with the anti-instinctual forces available to consciousness in the preconscious level of the mind.

These new factors, the importance of which were gradually borne in on Freud out of his increasing clinical experience over the years, were of critical significance. They ultimately led him to discard the topographic theory, to the extent that it was concerned with the assessment of specific processes related to specific regions of the mind. More precisely, Freud came to realize that what is more important is whether these processes belong to the primary system or the secondary system. The divisions of the mind into unconscious, preconscious, and conscious levels of functioning were not adequate to account for the broader spectrum of clinical data. The concepts that were part of this earlier theory and that have retained their usefulness refer to the characteristics of primary and secondary thought processes, the essential importance of wish fulfillment, and the tendency toward regression under conditions of frustration or stress, and finally, the existence of a dynamic unconscious and the nature of its operation.

From Topographic to Structural Perspective

The germination of the shifting currents of Freud's thinking finally came to fruition in his abandoning the topographic model and replacing it with the structural model of the psychic apparatus. The structural model was finally formulated and presented in *The Ego and the Id*, published in 1923. The introduction of the structural hypothesis initiated a new era in psychoanalytic thinking. The structural model of the mind, or the "tripartite theory" as it is often called, was composed of three distinct entities or organizations within the psychic apparatus—the id, the ego, and the superego.

The terms have become so familiar and the tendency to hypostatize them so great that it is well to bear in mind their nature as scientific constructs. The terms are theoretical constructs that have as their primary referents the specific mental functions and operations that they are intended to organize and integrate into higher order systems. Each refers to a particular aspect of mental functioning, and no one of them expresses or represents the sum total of mental functioning at any one time. If they often function as quasi-independent systems, they are, nonetheless, ultimately coordinated aspects of the operation of the mental apparatus. Moreover, unlike such phenomena as infantile sexuality or object relations, id, ego, and superego are not empirically demonstrable phenomena in themselves but must be inferred from the observable effects of the operations of specific psychic functions.

It should be noted that the functional view of the systemic approach to ego psychology, which was responsible for much of the elaboration and systematization of the thinking about the ego and its functions, treats the ego as "an organization of functions." This functional view presents the ego as an impersonal system composed of functions, thus giving the ego a highly mechanized and impersonal referent. This view is troublesome to some theorists because the functional view bypasses and leaves open to question the role in psychoanalytic theory of the introspectively grasped, subjective experience of self. The objection is that the systematic and functional view of the ego seems to rule out of psychoanalytic theory the human person as the subjective source of action and behavior. This problem, discussed later, remains a basic one for psychoanalytic thinking even today.

Many writers have commented that Freud's attention was directed to the structural aspects of the mind and the functioning of the ego at a relatively late stage in the development of psychoanalysis. In fact, the structural concepts underwent a gradual evolution in the course of Freud's thinking. Careful review of even early formulations reveals that he clearly associated certain aspects of mental functioning with characteristics of the mind, which were only synthesized and attributed to structural mental entities with the formulation of the structural theory. In general, those aspects of the mind that he regarded as responsible in one way or another for the repressive activity of the mind were later seen to be attributable to the structural ego and superego. The censor, for example in dream theory, was a mental entity that carried the burden of certain ego and superego functions, but was never explicitly recognized as a structural mental entity.

During the years of his early discoveries, however, Freud was interested primarily in establishing the existence of unconscious mental processes and in elucidating their nature. Concomitantly, he concerned himself with demonstrating the value of psychoanalysis as a potential technique for exploring the depths of the human mind. There is little surprise, then, that he would be less concerned with a detailed study of aspects of mental functioning that are normally more or less accessible to consciousness. Many of these aspects were already the object of psychological inquiry. The end of the 19th century saw the founding and early flourishing of experimental approaches to psychology. Only when Freud discovered that not all unconscious processes could be attributed merely to the instincts, that certain aspects of mental functioning associated with repressive activity were also unconscious as well, was he forced to turn to a more careful delineation and study of these mental structural components.

Historical Development of Ego Psychology

The evolution of the concept of ego within the framework of the historical development of psychoanalytic theory parallels to a large extent the shifts in Freud's view of the instincts and, following Rapaport, can be divided into four phases. The first phase ended in 1897 and coincided with the development of the early psychoanalytic formulations. The second phase extended from 1897 to 1923, thus spanning the development of psychoanalysis proper. The third phase, from 1923 to 1937, saw the development of Freud's theory of the ego and the gradual emergence to prominence of the ego in the overall context of the theory. Parallel to this development was the evolution of Freud's thinking about anxiety. Finally, the fourth phase, coming after Freud's death, saw the emergence and systematic development of a general psychology of the ego at the hands of Hartmann, Kris, Rapaport, and their followers, as well as a shifting of focus from the operation of ego functions themselves to the broader social and cultural contexts within which the ego developed and functioned, particularly following the lead of Erik Erikson.

First Phase: Early Concepts of the Ego

In the initial phase of the development of psychoanalytic theory, the ego was not always precisely defined. Rather, it referred to the dominant mass of conscious ideas and moral values, which were distinct from the impulses and wishes of the repressed unconscious. Thus, the ego was considered to be concerned primarily with defense, a term

Freud soon replaced with the notion of repression. At this stage repression and defense were regarded as synonymous. In the neurophysiological jargon of the *Project*, the ego was described as "an organization . . . whose presence interferes with passages [of quantity (of excitation)]" (1 *SE* 323). Translating this into the language of psychology, as in *Studies on Hysteria* or *The Interpretation of Dreams*, the ego was regarded as an agent that erected a defense against certain ideas that were unacceptable to consciousness. These ideas were found to be primarily sexual in nature and were initially thought to have been engendered by premature sexual trauma and real seduction. Presumably, because the memory of such trauma led to the arousal of unpleasant and painful affects, they evoked a defensive response and a repression of the original thought content. This repression, however, led to a damming up of energy and the consequent production of anxiety. The functioning of this "early ego" was contradictory to a degree because its primary purpose was to reduce tension and thus avoid unpleasant affects connected with sexual thoughts, but in the process of repression it seemed to evoke an equally unpleasant affect state, that of anxiety.

It is important to note the role of reality in this early theory. Until 1897, it was Freud's firm belief that the accounts of traumatic sexual experiences provided by his patients as memories of early childhood experiences were in fact real traumata. He envisioned the task of the ego as one of warding off the memories of these events. The ego was motivated in this task by considerations involving the individual's relationship with the real world or, more accurately, with the ideational representations of real experiences. With the collapse of the seduction hypothesis, however, the investigation of this aspect of ego functioning receded into the background. The focus was on internal, instinctually derived, and fantasy-dominated experience. The role of reality in the influencing of behavior was minimized. It is only recently, with the increasing interest in ego psychology, that the important role of the ego in mediating the individual's relationship with the outside world of events and human relationships has become a focus of increasing concern and study once again. The role of reality has particularly reasserted itself in relation to the vicissitudes of object relations in connection with the capacity for and development of ego functioning. It shall be seen, however, that the implications of reality and its role in psychoanalytic thinking are considerably broader.

Second Phase: Historical Roots of Ego Psychology

The score and more of years that preceded the publication of *The Ego and the Id* were dedicated to the development of psychoanalysis proper. During this period the analysis of the ego as such received little direct attention because Freud was concerned primarily with the instinctual drives, their representatives, and their transformations. Consequently, references to defense or to defensive functions were much less frequent. As indicated, there were areas of confusion and contradiction in Freud's early theory of the instincts and in his more limited topographic conception of the mind. The clarification of these concepts required further elucidation of the ego, its functions, and the nature of its organization. It was during this second phase that Freud grappled with these problems and gradually approached the more definitive resolution provided by the structural theory.

In regard to the sexual instinct, in 1915 in his "Instincts and Their Vicissitudes," Freud discussed the vicissitudes to which instincts were subjected as they sought expression. These vicissitudes included: reversal into its opposite (a sadistic impulse might be changed to a masochistic impulse), turning on the subject's own self (the love for the object might be turned toward the self), repression, or, finally, the instinct might be subjected to sublimation. When they are approached from the standpoint of the ego, each of these vicissitudes might be viewed as a defense mechanism. The ego's relationship to reality is particularly relevant in this connection. As noted earlier, the concept of a secondary process implies the ability to delay discharge of the instinctual drives in accordance with the demands of external reality. The capacity for delay was later to be ascribed to the ego. The progression from pleasure principle to reality principle in childhood involves a similar capacity to "postpone gratification" and thereby conform to the requirements of the outside world. The important relationship of libido to the self, as was postulated in the theory of narcissism, calls for a clearer understanding of the self, which in this phase has not yet been completely defined. According to the topographic theory of the mind, the preconscious, which by definition was accessible to consciousness, was held responsible for censorship. In many instances, however, this was an unconscious operation, thereby requiring a new formulation of the agency performing this function. Another problem arose in relation to the ego or self-preservative instincts held responsible for repression: presumably, the instincts were responsible for defense, but surely this task also belonged to the ego.

Finally, if neither the preconscious nor the ego instincts were solely responsible for repression or censorship, how was repression to be achieved? Freud tried to answer this question by postulating that ideas are maintained in the unconscious by a withdrawal of libido or energy (cathexis). In the manner characteristic of unconscious ideas, however, they constantly renew their attempt to become attached to libido and thus reach consciousness. Consequently, the withdrawal of libido must be constantly repeated. Freud described this process as "anticathexis" or "countercathexis." Again, however, if such countercathexis is to be consistently effective against unconscious ideas, it must be permanent and must itself operate on an unconscious basis. Understanding of psychic structure, specifically of the ego, which could perform this complicated function, was clearly called for and constituted still another indication of the need for the development of ego psychology. Thus, the way was pointed toward the third phase, wherein the ego was delineated as a structural entity and separated definitively from the instinctual drives.

Third Phase: Freud's Ego Psychology

With publication of *The Ego and the Id* in 1923, the phase of the introduction and development of Freud's own theory of the ego was accomplished. The ego was presented as a structural entity, a coherent organization of mental processes and functions that was primarily organized around the perceptual-conscious system but also included structures responsible for resistance and unconscious defense. The ego at this stage was relatively passive and weak. Its functioning was still a resultant of the pressures deriving from id, superego, and reality. The ego was the helpless rider on the id's horse, more or less obliged to go where the id wished to go. The assumption remains that the ego is not only dependent on the forces of the id, but is somehow genetically derived and differentiated out of the id. Freud had as yet to recognize any real development of the ego comparable to the phases of libidinal development.

During this period the view of the ego underwent a radical transformation. Some of the details of this development were discussed in
connection with Freud's theory of anxiety. In *Inhibitions, Symptoms, and
Anxiety* in 1926, Freud repudiated the conception of ego as subservient
to the id. Signal anxiety became an autonomous function for the initiating of defense, and the capacity of the ego to turn passively experienced anxiety into active anticipation was underlined. Here, too, the
relatively rudimentary conception of the defensive capacity of the
ego was enlarged to include a variety of defenses that the ego had at its
disposal and could utilize in the control and direction of id impulses.
Moreover, the elaboration of Freud's conception of the reality principle introduced a function of adaptation that allowed the ego to curb
instinctual drives when action prompted by them would lead into real
danger.

The effect of this transformation of his theory of the ego was three-
fold. First, it brought the ego into prominence as a powerful regulatory force that was responsible for the integration and control of behavioral responses. Second, the role of reality was brought to center
stage in the theory of ego functioning. It had been banished to the
wings in the preceding quarter century, but the concern with the adaptive function of the ego again brought it back to prominence. Even so,
the conception of adaptation here was rudimentary and limited to the
ego's capacity to avoid danger. The notions that Freud was evolving
during this phase provided the foundation for the concept of the autonomy of the ego, which was to be developed by later theorists. Finally, it was toward the end of this period, particularly in his 1937
"Analysis, Terminable and Interminable," that Freud finally made explicit the assumption of independently inherited roots of the ego that
were quite independent of the inherited roots of the instinctual drives.
This formulation was taken over by Hartmann and was the basis for
his notion of primary ego autonomy, which consequently stimulated
the developments of the fourth phase.

Fourth Phase: The Systematization of Ego Psychology

If the third phase can be thought of as culminating in Anna Freud's
work on the defense mechanisms of the ego, the fourth phase can be
seen as taking its initiation from the publication of Heinz Hartmann's

work on the ego and adaptation. Hartmann's work primarily focused on two aspects of Freud's later notions of the ego; namely, the autonomy of the ego and the problem of adaptation. The discussion of the apparatuses of primary autonomy was the basis for a doctrine of the genetic roots of the ego and a development of the notion of epigenetic maturation. Hartmann's treatment of adaptation also brought the adaptational point of view into focus in such a way that it has become generally acceptable as one of the basic metapsychological assumptions of psychoanalytic theory.

The adaptational approach, however, also served a broader purpose; namely, the consolidation of psychoanalysis as a general psychology, one which could communicate with, assimilate, and theoretically integrate the experimental and clinical study of psychological phenomena from other allied scientific disciplines involved in the study of human behavior. One of the important consequences, therefore, of Hartmann's work was that the concentration on and elaboration of the theory of the ego gradually enlarged the comprehension of ego functioning in such a way that other aspects of the tripartite theory were somewhat shunted aside and given only minor consideration. The process has been referred to as "egotization" of psychoanalysis.

Although the development of thinking about the ego was an important advance, many psychoanalysts began to feel that it created an imbalance in the theory and that, by increasingly focusing on the mechanical and quantitative aspects of ego functioning, it left a picture of personality functioning and dysfunctioning that seemed relatively inhuman. Moreover, as the process of egotization took place, there developed a widening split between the id, the vital stratum of the mind and the dynamic source of psychic energies, and the noninstinctual, nondynamic, structural apparatuses of the ego. Consequently, the id increasingly came to be seen as the source of instinctual energies—the image of the seething cauldron—without the representational or directional qualities that so long characterized Freud's views of the instincts and their functions.

The other extremely important aspect of the fourth phase is the reemergence of the importance of reality in its broadest and most profound meanings as a significant dimension of psychoanalytic thinking. This is in many ways a direct extrapolation of Hartmann's thinking about adaptation, because the adaptive functioning of the organism has directly to do with its fitting in with the requirements of external reality and adaptively interacting with the environment, not only the inanimate, but also the personal and social environment.

The concern with reality has led in two important directions. The first is the work of Erik Erikson, who has posed the question of the adaptation of the personality through the whole of the life cycle. He has reviewed this progressive elaboration and integration of personality as the resolution of life crises, as a progressive problem of adaptation to and resolution of the characteristic conflicts and crises that arise at various phases of human experience from birth to death. Thus, in Erikson's thinking, not merely the human environment, in which the human organism develops and with which it interacts, but also the broader reaches of the social and cultural environment have taken on an increasing importance in psychoanalytic perspective.

The other important extension of the principle of adaptation has been in the direction of object relations theory. The major focus of concern for the object relations school has been the interaction between the child and the important figures who people the child's early environment and who give decisive direction to the child's personality development. The emphasis in the object relations approach to the source of psychopathology is on the deficiencies of the environment—rather than on the internal vicissitudes of the instincts—or on more constitutional defects that would impair the course of development. An important consideration in thinking about the contributions of the object relations theorists is that, for the most part, their theoretical concerns derive from their unique patient population, which consists primarily of character disorders and forms of personality organization that are somewhat more primitive and show deeper levels of ego defect than the types of psychoneurotic patients traditionally dealt with in psychoanalysis.

Structure of the Psychic Apparatus

One of the current leading concerns of psychoanalytic theorists has to do with the integration of these more recent approaches with traditional psychoanalytic theory. Thus, the following more or less systematic survey of the tripartite theory is seen from the contemporary perspective, rather than from the historical perspective of the third phase. From a structural viewpoint, the psychic apparatus is divided into three provinces designated as id, ego, and superego. They are distinguished by their different functions. The main distinction lies between the ego and id. The id is the locus of the instinctual drives and is under the domination of the primary process. It operates according to the dictates of the pleasure principle, without regard for the limiting demands of reality. The ego, however, represents a coherent organization of functions, the task of which is to avoid unpleasure or pain by opposing or regulating the discharge of instinctual drives to conform to the demands of the external world. The regulation of id discharges is also contributed to by a third structural component of the psychic apparatus, the superego, which contains the internalized moral values, prohibitions, and standards of the parental imagos.

The Id

Freud separated the instinctual drives in his tripartite theory into a separate province, the vital stratum of the mind, and in so doing reached the culminating point of the evolution of his theory of instincts, as has been seen. Freud borrowed the term "id" from Georg Groddeck, an internist who became a somewhat enthusiastic apostle of the unconscious and first used the term in his own *The Book of the Id*. Originally, the term stood for all that was ego-alien. In contrast to his concept of the ego as an organized, problem-solving agent, Freud conceived of the id as a completely unorganized, primordial reservoir of energy, derived from the instincts, that is under the domination of the primary process. It was not, however, synonymous with the unconscious, because the structural viewpoint was unique in that it demonstrated that certain functions of the ego, specifically certain defenses against unconscious instinctual pressures, were unconscious; for the most part the superego itself also operated on an unconscious level.

Freud postulated that the id was primarily a hereditary given, such that the infant at birth was endowed with an id with instinctual drives seeking gratification. The infant has no capacity to delay, control, or modify these drives. Consequently, in the beginning of life, the infant is completely dependent on the egos of the caretaking persons in its environment to enable it to cope with the external world.

Although the segregation of instinctual drives in the id had the advantage of resolving certain observational and theoretical difficulties, it also left a residue of problems. Perhaps the most significant problem is that, in having separated the instincts, Freud left to the subsequent generations of psychoanalytic theorists the problem of dealing with ways in which instinctual components were effectively integrated with the functioning of the structural aspects of the psychic apparatus. The problem in many respects remains today and has become a focus of much contemporary controversy in psychoanalytic circles.

The other important problem that this separation left to be dealt with was the question of how much structure is involved in the functioning of the id. The tendency among systematic ego theorists has been to reduce the id progressively to simple energic forces with a minimum of structure. This is the correlative aspect of the tendency to regard all organization or representational functioning as related to the ego. Freud, however, was quite clear that the instinctual drives of the id had a vectorial and representational component and that they were organized according to the primary process, which is not a process of random discharge but is, in fact, a modality of organization. The question of the characteristics and degree of id organization is one on which psychoanalytic theorists differ and one that remains an unresolved theoretical issue.

Partly in an attempt to resolve some of these difficulties, Hartmann and his followers proposed that the id and the ego did not have separate origins, but that they both developed out of an undifferentiated matrix present at birth and that the separation into separate provinces, defined as id and ego, was a function of the developmental process.

The Ego

It was pointed out earlier in this discussion that those conscious and preconscious functions typically associated with the ego—for example, words, ideas, or logic—did not account entirely for its role in mental functioning. The discovery that certain phenomena that emerge most clearly in the psychoanalytic treatment setting, specifically repression and resistance, which were associated with the ego, could themselves be unconscious pointed up the need for an expanded concept of the ego as an organization retaining original close relationship to consciousness and to external reality and yet performing a variety of unconscious operations in relationship to the drives and their regulation. Once the scope of the ego had been thus broadened, consciousness was redefined as a mental quality that, although exclusive to the ego, constitutes only one of its qualities or functional aspects, rather than a separate mental system itself.

No more comprehensive definition of the ego is available than the one Freud provided toward the end of his career in 1938 in his *Outline of Psychoanalysis:*

> *Here are the principal characteristics of the ego.* In consequence of the pre-established connection between sense and perception and muscular action, the ego has voluntary movement at its command. It has the task of self-preservation. As regards *external* events, it performs that task by becoming aware of stimuli, by storing up experiences about them (in the memory), by avoiding excessively strong stimuli (through flight), by dealing with moderate stimuli (through adaptation) and finally by learning to bring about expedient changes in the external world to its own advantage (through activity). As regards *internal* events, in relation to the id, it performs that task by gaining control over the demands of the instinct, by deciding whether they are to be allowed satisfaction, by postponing that satisfaction to times and circumstances favourable in the external world or by suppressing their excitations entirely. It is guided in its activity by consideration of the tension produced by stimuli, whether these tensions are present in it or introduced into it. [23 *SE* 145–146]

Thus, the ego controls the apparatus of motility and perception, contact with reality, and, through the mechanisms of defense, the inhibition of primary instinctual drives.

Origins of the Ego

If the ego is defined as a coherent system of functions for mediating between the instincts and the outside world, one must concede that the newly born infant has no ego or, at best, the most rudimentary of egos. As previously noted, the neonate certainly has a rather complex array of capacities and both sensory and motor functions. There is, however, little coherent organization of these, so that one must say that the ego is at best rudimentary. Developmental ego psychology is then faced with the problem of explaining the processes that permit modification of the id and the concomitant genesis of the ego.

Freud believed that the modification of the id occurs as a result of the impact of the external world on the drives. The pressures of external reality enable the ego to appropriate the energies of the id to do its work. In the process of formation, the ego seeks to bring the influences of the external world to bear on the id, substitute the reality principle for the pleasure principle, and thereby contribute to its own further development. In summary, Freud emphasized the role of the instincts in ego development and, particularly, the role of conflict. At first this conflict is between the id and the outside world, but later it is between the id and the ego itself.

The work of Heinz Hartmann and his collaborators has expanded and modified this theory. Hartmann postulated the existence of primary autonomous ego functions, the development of which is independent of the drives and of conflicts. Specifically, Hartmann, Kris, and Loewenstein have suggested that the ego does not differentiate from the id, as such, but that both develop from a common undifferentiated matrix. It follows that the rudimentary apparatuses underlying the primary autonomous ego functions, such as perception, motility, memory, and intelligence, are present from birth. This concept further implies that there may be congenital or genetically determined variations in ego functions. This hypothesis was actually advanced by Freud in 1937, but it was greatly expanded and elaborated by Hartmann over a score of years, thus providing a more solid footing for his emerging concepts of ego autonomy. The elaboration of this view also contributed a genetic viewpoint to the theory of ego development.

In addition, Hartmann also elaborated the role of rudimentary ego apparatuses in the infant's coordinations with the object and the environment for the satisfaction of instinctual needs and drives. These early coordinations are the basis for Hartmann's development of the adaptive functions of the ego; that is, the function as mediator between external reality and the needs and demands of other psychic systems— id and superego. The adaptive functions of the ego are related to Hartmann's concept of ego development. The optimal functioning of the

organism requires a balance of these controlling forces—ego autonomy from the demands of the id, as well as ego autonomy from the demands of the environment.

Development of the Ego

The processes by which the internal world is built up and by which
structure is consolidated within the self are referred to under the heading of internalization. Forms of internalization—incorporation, introjection, and identification—are variously connected with development
of the ego.

Incorporation

Incorporation was originally conceived of as an instinctual activity
derived from and based on the oral phase and was considered as a genetic precursor of identification. However, even though incorporation
fantasies are often associated with internalizing processes, they are by
no means identical and may be quite independent. Some authors have
envisioned incorporation as the mechanism of primary identification,
aimed at a primary union between oneself and the maternal object.

Incorporation as a mechanism of internalization seems to involve
a primitive oral wish for union with an object. The union has a quality
of totality and globalization, so that in the internalization of the object, the object loses all distinction and function as object. The external
object is completely assumed into the person's inner world. Incorporation is thus operative in relatively regressive conditions. Incorporation is the most primitive, least differentiated form of internalization,
in which the object loses its distinction as object and becomes totally
assumed into the person's inner world, so that self and object are experienced as one. Consequently, incorporation has little to do with ego
development.

Introjection

Perhaps the most central process in the development of the structural apparatus, that is, id, ego, and superego, is the process of introjection. Introjection was originally described by Freud in "Mourning
and Melancholia" as a process of narcissistic identification in which
the lost object is introjected and thus retained as a part of the internal
structure of the psyche. Freud later applied this mechanism to the

genesis of the superego, making introjection the primary internalizing mechanism by which parental imagoes are internalized at the close of the oedipal phase. The child tries to retain the gratifications derived from these object relationships, at least in fantasy, through the process of introjection. By this mechanism, qualities of the person who was the center of the gratifying relationship are internalized and reestablished as part of the organization of the self. Freud referred to this internalized product as a "precipitate of abandoned object cathexis."

The basic parameters of Freud's original formulation are still applicable—namely, that the mechanism implies abandonment of an object relation and the preservation of the lost object intrapsychically by way of internalization, which is defensively motivated and expressive of basic instinctual determinants, especially aggressive and narcissistic.

The introject comes to exercise a particular influence on a person's inner state and behavior, and the relationships between the person and the introject are as varied as the relationships between two persons. The introject is the inner presence of an external object. Such a "presence" can be recognized only when it becomes conscious, but it may be active and effective when unconscious or subconscious. As a quasi-active presence, then, the introject provides a structural means for binding and integrating basic instinctual energies.

The introject must be regarded as a quasi-autonomous source of intrapsychic influence and activity that can substitute for the lost object as a source of narcissistic gratification or even aggressive impulse. The effect of the introject is to modify the self, so that it acquires characteristics of the internalized object. The introject is, therefore, a center of functional organization, possessing its own relative autonomy in the economy of psychic function. Because of their tendency to regression and their susceptibility to instinctual influences, introjects must be considered as more structuralizing than structured, more feeble, less stable, and more transient than the less instinctually derived, secondary process organization of more autonomous identificatory systems.

Identification
Identification has often been confused with introjection, partially because the two processes were treated in an overlapping and

somewhat interchangeable fashion by Freud. There are, nonetheless, grounds for maintaining a distinction between them. Identification is, properly speaking, an active structuralizing process that takes place within the self, by which the ego constructs the inner constituents of regulatory control on the basis of selected elements derived from the model. What constitutes the model of identification can vary considerably and can include introjects, structural aspects of real objects, or even value components of group structures and group cultures. The process of identification is specifically an intrasystemic structuralizing activity, attributed to the ego, related to its synthetic function and affecting structural integration in all parts of the psychic apparatus, including superego.

The lines that differentiate identification from introjection should be kept clear. Introjection operates as a function of instinctual forces—both libidinal and aggressive—so that in conjunction with projection it functions intimately in the vicissitudes of instinctual motivation and derivatives. Identification, however, functions relatively autonomously from instinctual derivatives. Introjection is indirectly involved in the transformation and binding of basic motivation influences. Hence, introjection is much more influenced by these derivatives, and its binding permits greater susceptibility to regressive pulls and to primary process forms of organization. The result of integration through identification, however, is more autonomous, more resistant to regressive pulls, and organized more specifically in secondary process terms. Identification, therefore, is the mechanism for the formation of structures of secondary autonomy.

Both introjection and identification are involved in the formation of structure. Introjection is directly involved in the formation of structural modifications within the self. Nevertheless, the introjective nuclei that constitute the core of the superego intrinsically modify psychic structure but do not directly affect ego structure as such. Identifications, however, are directly and specifically structural modifications attributed, as such, and integrated into the ego core of the personality.

Thus, both processes play a role in the development of the psychic apparatus, but their functions are quite distinct. Introjection is taken up in the working through of instinctual vicissitudes; identification is specifically involved primarily in the development of ego structures and functions and secondarily in development within the self as a whole. Development must be seen as a complex process in which introjection and identification are continually interacting with intrinsic maturational factors—introjection interacting more explicitly with instinctual factors and identification more with ego factors. Both are likewise subject to the laws of epigenesis, but they differ in their patterns of primacy—introjection exercising its developmental influence predominantly earlier in the course of development and identification assuming increasing importance in later phases of development.

Functions of the Ego

This discussion of ego functions is based on the preceding definition of the ego as a substratum of personality, comprising an organization of functions that share in common the task of mediating between the instincts and the outside world. Thus, the ego is a subsystem of the personality and is not synonymous with the self, the personality, or character.

Any attempt to draw up a complete list of ego functions would have to be relatively arbitrary. Invariably, the list of basic ego functions suggested by various authors differs in varying degrees. This discussion will be limited to several functions generally conceded to be fundamental to ego operation.

Control and Regulation of Instinctual Drives

The development of the capacity to delay immediate discharge of urgent wishes and impulses is essential if the ego is to assure the integrity of the individual and fulfill its role as mediator between the id and the outside world. The development of the capacity to delay or postpone instinctual discharge, like the capacity to test reality, is closely related to the progression in early childhood from the pleasure principle to the reality principle.

The progression from pleasure to reality principle parallels the development of secondary process (or logical) thinking, which aids in the control of drive discharge. The evolution of thought, from the initially prelogical primary process thinking to the more logical and deliberate secondary process thinking, is one of the means by which the ego learns to postpone the discharge of instinctual drives. For example, the representation in fantasy of instinctual wishes as fulfilled may obviate the need for urgent action, which might not always serve the realistic needs of the individual. Similarly, the capacity to "figure things out" or anticipate consequences represents thought processes essential to the realistic functioning of the individual. Obviously, the ego's capacity to control instinctual life and to regulate thinking is closely associated with its defensive functioning.

In this connection, it is important to highlight the role of the ego in the use of signal affects as part of its adaptive repertoire. Freud's original notion, derived from the second theory of anxiety, has been enlarged to extend to a variety of signal affects. Thus, it seems clear that the ego can use the affects of anxiety and depression as signals of instinctual or other danger and may also have other affective states that it can exploit in the same manner—including possibly guilt and shame—as the means of adaptively mobilizing defensive capacities. The essential notion is that the ego is partly in the position of exploiting the instinctual impulses as a means of organizing anticipatory signals, which then elicit more effective defensive alignments to prevent the disruptive and overwhelming breakthrough of threatening instinctual contents. It should be noted that the signal function of such affective states is not only in the service of mobilizing defense but is, as previously noted, an essential part of the ego's emerging capacity to tolerate pain and frustration; thus they contribute to the building up and maintenance of structural apparatuses that, in turn, contribute to the regulation of instinctual drives. It is not yet clear what the relationship of this utilization of secondary or signal anxiety is to the internalizing processes discussed above, but it may be that the toleration of moderate amounts of anxiety or other dysphoric affects within manageable and relatively less threatening limits minimizes the defensive interference of introjective configurations and allows for the relatively nonconflictual and independent operation of ego-consolidating identifications and other synthetic processes.

Relation to Reality

Freud always regarded the ego's capacity for maintaining relationship to the external world among its principal functions. The character of its relationship to the external world may be divided into three components: (1) the sense of reality, (2) reality testing, and (3) the adaptation to reality.

Sense of Reality.   The sense of reality originates simultaneously with the development of the ego. Infants first become aware of the reality of their own bodily sensations. Only gradually do they develop the capacity to distinguish a reality outside of their own bodies.

Reality Testing.   This refers to the ego's capacity for objective evaluation and judgment of the external world, which depends first on the primary autonomous functions of the ego, such as memory and perception, but then also on the relative integrity of internal structures of secondary autonomy. Under conditions of internal stress, in which regressive pulls are effectively operating, introjective aspects of the inner psychic structure can tend to dominate and, thus, become susceptible to projective distortions that color the individual's perception and interpretation of the outside world. Because of the fundamental importance of reality testing for "negotiating" with the outside world, its impairment may be associated with severe mental disorder. The development of the capacity to test reality, which is closely related to the progression from pleasure principle to reality principle, or to distinguish fantasy from actuality, occurs gradually. This capacity, once gained, is subject to regression and temporary deterioration in children, even up to school age, in the face of anxiety, conflict, intense instinctual wishes, or developmental crisis. This is not to be confused, however, with the breakdown of reality testing referred to above, which occurs in adult forms of psychopathology.

Adaptation to Reality.   This function refers to the capacity of the ego to use the individual's resources to form adequate solutions based on previously tested judgments of reality. It is possible for the ego to develop not only good reality testing, with perception and grasp, but also to develop an adequate capacity to accommodate the individual's resources to the situation thus perceived. Adaptation is closely allied to the concept of mastery, both in respect to external tasks and to the instincts. It should be distinguished from adjustment, which may entail accommodation to reality at the expense of certain resources or potentialities of the individual. The function of adaptation to reality is closely related to the defensive functions of the ego. The mechanism that may serve defensive purposes from one point of view may simultaneously serve adaptive purposes when viewed from another perspective. Thus, in the obsessive-compulsive person, intellectualization may serve important inner needs to control drive impulses, but by the same token, from another perspective the intellectual activity itself may be serving highly adaptive functions in dealing with the complexities of external reality.

Object Relationships

The capacity for mutually satisfying relationships is one of the fundamental functions to which the ego contributes. Significance of object relationships and their disturbance—for normal psychological development and a variety of psychopathological states—was fully appreciated relatively late in the development of classical psychoanalysis. The evolution in the child's capacity for relationships with others, which progresses from narcissism to social relationships within the family and then to relationships within the larger community, has been described. Also, focus has been put on the early stages in the relationship to need satisfying and on the development of object constancy, which begins when the infant is about six months of age. The process of the development of object relationship may be disturbed by retarded development, regression, or conceivably by inherent genetic defects or limitations in the capacity to develop object relationships. The development of object relationships is closely related to the concomitant evolution of drive components and the phase-appropriate defenses that accompany them.

Defensive Functions of the Ego

It was pointed out previously that in his initial psychoanalytic formulations, and for a long time thereafter, Freud considered repression to be virtually synonymous with defense. More specifically, repression was directed primarily against the impulses, drives, or drive representations and, particularly, against direct expression of the sexual instinct. Defense was thus mobilized to bring instinctual demands into conformity with the demands of external reality. With the development of the structural view of the mind, the function of defense was ascribed to the ego. Only after Freud had formulated his final theory of anxiety, however, was it possible to study the operation of the various defense mechanisms in light of their mobilization in response to danger signals.

Thus, a systematic and comprehensive study of the defenses used by the ego was only presented for the first time by Anna Freud. In her classic monograph *The Ego and the Mechanisms of Defense* (1946), Anna Freud maintained that everyone, whether normal or neurotic, uses a characteristic repertoire of defense mechanisms, but to varying degrees. On the basis of her extensive clinical studies of children, she described their essential inability to tolerate excessive instinctual stimulation and discussed the processes whereby the primacy of such drives at various developmental stages evoked anxiety in the ego. This anxiety, in turn, produced a variety of defenses. With regard to adults, her psychoanalytic investigations led her to conclude that although resistance is an obstacle to progress in treatment, to the extent that it impedes the emergence of unconscious material, it also constitutes a useful source of information concerning the ego's defensive operations.

Genesis of Defense Mechanisms.   In the early stages of development, defenses emerge as a result of the ego's struggles to mediate the pressures of the id and the requirements and strictures of outside reality. At each phase of libidinal development, associated drive components evoke characteristic ego defenses. Thus, for example, introjection, denial, and projection are defense mechanisms that are associated with oral-incorporative or oral-sadistic impulses, whereas reaction formations, such as shame and disgust, usually develop in relation to anal impulses and pleasures. Defense mechanisms from earlier phases of development persist side by side with those of later periods. When defenses associated with pregenital phases of development tend to predominate in adult life over more mature mechanisms, such as sublimation and repression, the personality retains an infantile cast.

The repertoire that an individual characteristically uses to deal with stress-evoking situations makes an important contribution to character formation. Character traits, such as excessive orderliness, are closely related to defenses but are distinguished from them by their greater role both in the overall functioning of the personality and in situations that are not related to specific conflicts.

Although abnormalities in the development of the functioning of ego defenses, or defense mechanisms, may have a fundamental relationship to the etiology of various forms of psychopathology, defenses are not of themselves pathological. On the contrary, they may serve an essential function in maintaining normal psychological well-being. Nonetheless, psychopathology may arise as a result of one of a variety of possible alterations of normal defensive functioning. For example, in hysteria, the defense of repression is temporarily overwhelmed because of an excess of sexual stimulation. This revival of previously repressed wishes calls for more desperate and fragmented efforts at renewed repression, which themselves result in the formation of conversion or phobic symptoms. The individual, however, may show an exaggerated development and overuse of certain defenses, as if the danger posed by infantile sexual and aggressive impulses were as great in adult life as it was perceived to be in childhood. This kind of hypervigilance is characteristic of obsessive-compulsive neurotics.

Possibly the development of the ego and its defenses may itself be faulty, with excessive reliance placed on the denial-projection-distortion modes characteristic of early oral or narcissistic phases of development. In that event, the defense mechanisms, while permitting limited functioning, particularly in the original family setting that may share these defensive patterns, cannot adequately equip the adult to meet the challenges of the external world. Thus, they can impede the adult's capacity to form object attachments, to engage in heterosexual relationships, or to cope with vocational competition. When the defenses fail, there may be a breakthrough of direct instinctual expression and a regression in the ego's capacity to control instinctual motility. This breakthrough in defenses, and accompanying regression, is most graphically seen in states of acute schizophrenic turmoil.

Classification of Defenses.   It is possible to list the defenses used by the ego according to a variety of classifications, none of which is all-inclusive or takes into account all of the relevant factors. Defenses may be classified developmentally, for example, that is, in terms of the libidinal phase in which they arise. Thus, denial, projection, and distortion would be assigned to the oral stage of development and to the correlative narcissistic stage of object relationships. Certain defenses, however, such as magical thinking and regression, cannot be categorized in this way. Moreover, certain basic developmental processes, such as introjection and projection, may also serve defensive functions under certain specifiable conditions.

The defenses have also been classified on the basis of the particular form of psychopathology with which they are commonly associated. Thus, the obsessional defenses would include isolation, rationalization, intellectualization, and denial; however, defensive operations are not limited to pathological conditions. Finally, the defenses have been classified as to whether they are simple mechanisms or complex, in which a single defense would involve a combination or composite of simple mechanisms. Table B gives a brief classification and description of some of the basic defense mechanisms most frequently employed and most thoroughly investigated by psychoanalysts (see appendix).

Synthetic Function

The synthetic function of the ego, which was described by Nunberg in 1931, refers to the ego's capacity to integrate various aspects of its functioning. It involves the capacity of the ego to unite, organize, and bind together various drives, tendencies, and functions within the personality, enabling the individual to think, feel, and act in an organized and directed manner. Briefly, the synthetic function is concerned with the overall organization and functioning of the ego and consequently must enlist the cooperation of other ego functions in its operation.

Although the synthetic function subserves the interests of adaptive functioning in the ego, it may also bring together various forces in a way that, although not completely adaptive, is an optimal solution for the individual in a particular state at a given moment or period of time. Thus, the formation of a symptom that represents a compromise of opposing tendencies, although unpleasant in some degree, is nonetheless preferable to yielding to a dangerous instinctual impulse or, conversely, trying to stifle the impulse completely. Hysterical conversion, for example, combines a forbidden wish and the punishment for it into a physical symptom. On examination, the symptom often turns out to be the only possible compromise under the circumstances.

It should also be noted that the operation of the synthetic function is closely involved in the process of structure formation and integration during the course of development. Thus, the formation of introjects and their integration into progressive stages of personality development, as well as the even closer integration of identifications with the core sense of the self, can be seen in some part as a function of the ego's capacity for internal synthesis.

Autonomy of the Ego

Although Freud referred to "primal, congenital ego variations" as early as 1937, this concept was greatly expanded and clarified by Hartmann. As already observed in this discussion, Hartmann advanced a basic formulation about development; that is, that the ego and id differentiate from a common matrix, the so-called undifferentiated phase, in which the ego's precursors are inborn apparatuses of primary autonomy. These apparatuses are rudimentary in nature, present at birth, and develop outside the area of conflict with the id. This area Hartmann referred to as a "conflict-free" area of ego functioning. He included perception, intuition, comprehension, thinking, language, certain phases of motor development, learning, and intelligence among the functions in this "conflict-free" sphere. Each of these functions, however, might also become involved in conflict secondarily in the course of development. For example, if aggressive, competitive impulses intrude on the impulse to learn, they may evoke inhibitory defensive reactions on the part of the ego, thus interfering with the conflict-free operation of these functions.

Primary Autonomy

With the introduction of the primary autonomous structure of the ego, Hartmann introduced an independent genetic derivation for at least part of the ego, thus establishing it as an independent realm of psychic organization that was not totally dependent on and derived from the instincts and the intrinsic patterning of instinctual development. This was an insight of major importance because it laid the foundations for the emerging doctrine of ego autonomy and meant that the analysis of ego development would have to consider an entirely new set of variables quite separate from those involved in instinctual development.

It should be noted that this shift toward a consideration of autonomous factors followed a general functional tendency toward establishing psychoanalysis as a general psychology. Hartmann's emphasis was on the common factors that could be taken as underlying and influencing the process of development because he related the emergence of the primary autonomous factors to what he called the "average expectable environment." This reflected a trend toward generality in theory and a movement away from the focus on specific environmental factors, notably those embedded in the individual's object relationships, which were at work in the development of any given individual ego. This objection has been made not only about Hartmann's work but also about the whole systematic school of ego psychologists. Attempts to reverse and correct this abstractive tendency have been made recently with object relations theory.

Secondary Autonomy

Hartmann observed that the conflict-free sphere derived from the structures of primary autonomy can be enlarged, that further functions could be withdrawn from the domination of drive influences. This was Hartmann's concept of secondary autonomy. Thus, a mechanism that arose originally in the service of defense against instinctual drives may in time become an independent structure, such that the drive impulse merely triggers the automatized apparatus. Thus, the apparatus may come to serve other functions than the original defensive function, for example, adaptation or synthesis. Hartmann refers to this removal of specific mechanisms from drive influences as a process of change of function. It has often been observed that this process is akin to Gordon Allport's concept of functional autonomy.

Along with the development of the notion of autonomy, Hartmann also provided an economic basis for the support of autonomous functions. Obviously, the conflict-free functioning of these autonomous ego capacities could not be maintained on the basis of unmodified instinctual drives because the very notion of autonomy was to emphasize the withdrawal of these functions from drive influence. He thus proposed that at least some of the ego's energies may derive from non-drive sources; he also proposed the concept of neutralization as an alternate explanation for the energy utilized in conflict-free functions of the ego. Neutralization is a generalization of Freud's concept of sublimation or desexualization. *Neutralization* involves the desexualization of libidinal drives or the deaggressivization of aggressive drives and thus provides the ego with independent energies that function without drive interference or dependence. The extent to which instinctual energy becomes neutralized is a measure of ego-strength.

Hartmann makes it clear that all autonomy is relative. The ego may lose its autonomy if the drive influences increase disproportionately. Autonomy can also be diminished if synthetic functioning is weakened by toxic effects, the influence of illness, or even organic injuries. The loss or decompensation of defending or regulating structures can also lead to a process of deneutralization, so that instinctual drives come to influence the previously relatively autonomous functions. This may result in the undermining of secondary autonomous structures and can even influence the functioning of the apparatuses of primary autonomy. Such would be the case, for example, in hysterical blindness.

Although Hartmann envisioned autonomy in terms of the autonomy of the ego from the influence of the id, another aspect of autonomy was added by Rapaport in focusing on the autonomy of the ego from external reality. By this he meant the capacity of the psychic apparatus to respond in relative independence from external stimulation; that is, the ego's response capacity is not stimulus-bound. The autonomy of the ego had to be safeguarded from both influences. Rapaport wrote: "Thus, while the *ultimate guarantees of the ego's autonomy from the id* are man's constitutionally given apparatuses of reality relatedness, the *ultimate guarantees of the ego's autonomy from the environment* are man's constitutionally given drives" (1967:727).

Thus, although the appreciation of the autonomy in function and structure of the ego from drive and environmental influences was a major contribution of the systematic ego school, there remain significant difficulties that need to be resolved. One of the important areas for thinking and investigation in psychoanalysis has to do with the influences and determining factors of the development of ego autonomy. One of the major areas of theoretical tension has to do with the

emergence of autonomous functions and autonomous ego structures, along with the understanding of both their removal from and
their involvement in instinctual sources of energy. There is a tendency
in this area to follow Hartmann's lead in the direction of postulating
independent sources of ego-energy—independent, that is, from instinctual sources. This tendency, however, raises the further problem of resolving and integrating the instinctual and the independent
ego-energies in the course of development of an integrated psychic
apparatus.

The Superego

The origins and functions of the superego are to a significant degree
involved with those of the ego, but they reflect different developmental
vicissitudes. Briefly, the superego is the last of the structural components to develop, resulting from the resolution of the oedipal complex.
As previously mentioned, it is concerned with moral behavior based on
unconscious behavioral patterns learned at early pregenital stages of
development.

The structural model provides a useful means of expressing the
nature of neurotic conflict. Neurotic conflict can be explained structurally as a conflict between the forces of the ego, on one hand, and the
forces of the id, on the other. Frequently, the superego participates in
the conflict by allying itself with the ego and thus imposing demands
in the form of conscience or guilt feelings. Occasionally, however, the
superego may be allied with the id against the ego. This happens in
cases of severely regressed reaction, where the functions of the superego may become sexualized once more or may become permeated by
aggression, taking on a quality of primitive (usually anal) destructiveness, thus reflecting the quality of the instinctual drives in question.

Historical Development

The concept of the superego, like the ego, has its historical origins
in Freud's writings. The steps leading up to its formulations as a special
agency of the mind can be traced to a paper written in 1896, "Further
Remarks on the Neuro-Psychoses of Defense," in which he described
obsessional ideas as "*self-reproaches* which have re-emerged from *re-*

pression and which always relate to some *sexual* act that was performed with pleasure in *childhood*" (3 *SE* 169).

The activity of a self-criticizing agency is also implicit in Freud's early discussions of dreams, which postulate the existence of a "censor" that does not permit unacceptable ideas to enter consciousness on moral grounds.

He first discussed the concept of a special self-critical agency in 1914, when he published his exposition of narcissism. In "On Narcissism," Freud suggested that a hypothetical state of narcissistic perfection existed in early childhood; at this stage, the child was his or her own ideal. As the child grew up, the admonitions of others and self-criticism combined to destroy this perfect image. To compensate for this lost narcissism, or to recover it, the child "projects before him" a new ideal, or ego-ideal. It was at this point that Freud suggested that the psychic apparatus might have still another structural component, a special agency whose task it was to watch over the ego, to make sure it was measuring up to the ego-ideal. The concept of the superego evolved from these formulations of an ego-ideal and a second monitoring agency to ensure its preservation.

In the following year, 1915, in "Mourning and Melancholia," Freud speaks again of "one part of the ego" that "judges it critically and, as it were, takes it as its object" (14 *SE* 247). He suggests that this agency, which is split off from the rest of the ego, is what is commonly called conscience. He further states that this self-evaluating agency can act independently, become "diseased" on its own account, and should be regarded as a major institution of the ego. In 1921, Freud referred to this self-critical agency as the ego-ideal and held it responsible for the sense of guilt and for the self-reproaches typical in melancholia and depression. He had dropped his earlier distinction between the ego-ideal, or ideal self, and self-critical agency, or conscience.

In 1923, in *The Ego and the Id*, Freud's concept of the superego included both these functions; that is, the superego represented the ego-ideal as well as conscience. He also demonstrated that the operations of the superego were mainly unconscious. Thus, patients who were dominated by a deep sense of guilt lacerated themselves far more harshly on an unconscious level than they did consciously. The fact that guilt engendered by the superego might be eased by suffering or punishment was apparent in the case of neurotics who demonstrated an unconscious need for punishment. In later works Freud elaborated on the relationship between the ego and the superego. Guilt feelings were ascribed to tension between these two agencies, and the need for punishment was an expression of this tension.

In one of his last discussions of the superego, in *Civilization and Its Discontents* (1930), Freud expanded on its relationship to his evolving conception of the aggressive instinct: When an instinct undergoes repression, its libidinal aspects may be transformed into symptoms, whereas its aggressive components are transformed into a sense of guilt.

On another level Freud related the development of the superego to the evolution of culture and to the relation of human beings to one another in society. In such moral precepts as "Love thy neighbor," which are aimed at controlling aggression, the cultural superego makes demands on the individual from without, much as the personal superego dictates from within. Freud believed that the cultural superego, which represents the ideals of civilization, evolved from the impression left by the personalities of great leaders; that is, "men of overwhelming force of mind or men in whom one of the human impulsions has found its strongest and purest, and therefore often its most one-sided, expression" (21 *SE* 141).

Freud recognized that some limits on individual satisfactions were necessarily imposed by the demands of civilization, but he lamented deeply the degree to which the individual must renounce instinctual gratification to conform to the social requirements of the larger group. These ideas—which Freud posed very tentatively, recognizing that his application of individual psychology to society was merely by analogy—have been adopted and greatly extended, often on a rather superficial level, in various discussions of the neurotic culture of this century.

Origins of the Superego

The superego comes into being with the resolution of the Oedipus complex. During the oedipal period, the little boy wishes to possess his mother, the little girl wishes to possess her father. Each must, however, contend with a substantial rival, the parent of the same sex. The frustration of the child's positive oedipal wishes by this parent evokes intense hostility, which finds expression not only in overt antagonistic behavior but also in thoughts of killing the parent who stands in the way, along with any brothers or sisters who may also compete for the love of the desired parent.

Quite understandably, this hostility on the part of the child is unacceptable to the parent and, in fact, eventually becomes unacceptable to the child as well. In addition, the boy's sexual explorations and masturbatory activities may themselves meet with parental disfavor, which may even be underscored by real or implied threats of castration. These threats and, above all, the boy's observations that women and girls lack a penis convince him of the reality of castration. Consequently, he turns away from the oedipal situations and enters the latency period of psychosexual development. He renounces the sexual expressions of the infantile phase.

Girls, when they become aware of the fact that they lack a penis, that they have "come off badly," seek to redeem the loss by obtaining a penis or a baby from the father. Freud pointed out that although the anxiety surrounding castration brings the Oedipus complex to an end in boys, in girls it is the major precipitating factor. Girls renounce their oedipal strivings, first, because they fear the loss of the mother's love and, second, because of their disappointment over the father's failure to gratify their wish. The latency phase, however, is not so well-defined in girls as it is in boys, and their persistent interest in family relations is expressed in their play; throughout grade school, for example, girls "act out" the roles of wife and mother in games that boys scrupulously avoid.

Evolution of the Superego

What is, indeed, the fate of the object attachments that are given up with the resolution of the Oedipus complex? Freud's formulation of the mechanism of introjection is relevant here. During the oral phase, the child is entirely dependent on the parents. When advancing beyond this stage, the child must abandon the earliest symbiotic ties with the parents and form initial introjections of them, which, however, follow the anaclitic model; that is, they are characterized by dependence on another. The dissolution of the Oedipus complex and the concomitant abandonment of object ties lead to a rapid acceleration of the introjection process.

One might think, following the model proposed above, that the child would identify with the parent of the opposite sex after being forced to renounce oedipal object ties, and to some degree this may, in fact, occur. Under normal conditions, however, the striving toward masculinity in the boy and femininity in the girl leads to a stronger identification with the parent of the same sex. The problem is not simple; because of the bisexual potential of boys and girls, a child may emerge from the Oedipus complex with various admixtures of masculine and feminine introjections. Obviously, these introjections will have a great deal to do with ultimate character formation and later object choices.

With specific reference to superego formation, these introjections from both parents become united and form a kind of precipitate within the self, which then confronts the other contents of the psyche as a superego. This identification with the parents is based on the child's struggles to repress the instinctual aims that were directed toward them, and it is this effort of renunciation that gives the superego its prohibiting character. It is for this reason, too, that the superego results to such a great extent from an introjection of the parents' own superegos. Yet, because the superego evolves as a result of repression of the instincts, it has a closer relation to the id than does the ego itself. Its origins are more internal; the ego originates to a greater extent in the external world and is its representative.

Finally, throughout the latency period and thereafter, the child (and later the adult) continues to build on these early identifications through contact with teachers, heroic figures, and admired persons, who form the child's moral standards, values, and ultimate aspirations and ideals.

The child moves into the latency period endowed with a superego that is, as Freud put it, "the heir to the Oedipus complex" (23 *SE* 205). Its structures at first may be compared to the imperative nature of the demands of the id before it developed. The child's conflicts with the parents continue, of course, but now they are largely internal, between the ego and the superego. In other words, the standards, restrictions, commands, and punishments imposed previously by the parents from without are internalized in the child's superego, which now judges and guides behavior from within, even in the absence of the parents.

Clearly, this initially punitive superego must be modified and "softened," so that eventually it can permit adult sexual object choice and fulfillment. Adolescence poses a unique developmental hurdle in this regard. With the heightening of sexual and aggressive drives characteristic during this period, there is a threatened regressive revival of the abandoned incestuous ties to the parents and the undermining of the efforts of the superego. Often, the rebellious acting-out behavior of teenagers can be understood as instinctual release that the superego has failed to curb. Their behavior, however, may be deflected from the more threatening attachment to the parents to parental representatives beyond the familial world. In contrast, the superego of the ascetic, oversubmissive, or intellectual adolescent has responded to the threat posed by these heightened drives with renewed vigilance and intensified instinctual renunciation. The task of adolescence is to modify the oedipal identifications with the parents. Ideally, such modification will enable a love-object choice that is not motivated entirely by the need for a parent substitute or based exclusively on the need to rebel against their internalized imagos.

Current Investigations of the Superego

The exploration of the superego and its functions did not end with Freud, and such studies remain of active interest. Obviously, it is beyond the scope of this essay to discuss this work in detail. Recent interest, however, has focused on the difference between the superego and the ego-ideal, a distinction that Freud periodically revived and abandoned. Thus, at present, the term superego refers primarily to a self-critical, prohibiting agency bearing a close relationship to aggression and aggressive identifications. The ego-ideal, however, is a kinder agency, based on a transformation of the abandoned perfect state of narcissism, or self-love, which existed in early childhood and has been integrated with positive elements of identifications with the parents. In addition, the concept of an ideal object—that is, the idealized object choice—has been advanced as distinct from the ideal self. Many theorists regard the ego-ideal as an aspect of superego organization derived from good parental imagos.

A second focus of recent interest has been the contribution of the drives and object attachments formed in the preoedipal period to the development of the superego. These pregenital (especially anal) precursors of the superego are generally thought to provide the very rigid, strict, and aggressive qualities of the superego. These qualities stem from the projection of the child's own sadistic drives and primitive concept of justice based on retaliation, which was attributed to the parents during this period. The harsh emphasis on absolute cleanliness and propriety that is sometimes found in very rigid individuals and in obsessional neurotics is based to some extent on this sphincter morality of the anal period. Parenthetically, it should be noted that Melanie Klein's contention that the Oedipus complex, including the superego, is well established within the first year of life derives from another theoretical framework and is not to be confused with the concept of pregenital precursors of the superego, as postulated by classical psychoanalytic theory.

Metapsychological Assumptions

The metapsychological assumptions hold a special place in psychoanalytic theory. They consist of a set of basic assumptions or points of view that state the minimal (both necessary and sufficient) independent assumptions on which psychoanalytic theory rests. They may be regarded as the basic postulates or perspectives from which any given psychoanalytic proposition or any given segment of psychoanalytic theory must be viewed and interpreted. They can thus be regarded also as the most general propositions through which psychoanalytic thinking can be organized and integrated. Thus, in the order of increasing generality, in considering psychoanalytic theory one must take into account and distinguish between empirical propositions, specific psychoanalytic propositions, general propositions of psychoanalytic theory, and metapsychological assumptions. Metapsychological assumptions can be described in the following propositions.

The *economic point of view* has traditionally been conceptualized as psychological energies and their distribution and transformation. Thus, this point of view has been interpreted as the requirement that psychoanalytic explanation of any psychological phenomenon include propositions concerning psychological energies. It assumed, therefore, that psychological energies exist, follow a law of conservation, and are subject to the law of entropy (constancy, Nirvana). It also has assumed that these energies are subject to transformations that increase or decrease their entropic tendency.

The statement of the economic hypothesis in strictly energic terms seems no longer satisfactory or viable. The criticisms and difficulties with the concept of psychic energy have been discussed already, and there is no need to rehearse them here. It should be stressed, however, that the economic hypothesis as such does not rest on or require the notion of psychic energies, because this is at best a difficult and sometimes misleading metaphor. Any scientific account involving quantitative intensity, or even a theory allowing for degrees of structural complexity, stability, and levels of hierarchical organization, along with degrees of drive motility and structureless spontaneity, cannot function without at least an implicit principle of economics.

The *dynamic point of view* demands that the psychoanalytic explanation of any psychological phenomenon include propositions concerning psychological forces. It assumes that there are psychological forces defined by their direction and magnitude. The effect of simultaneously acting psychological forces may be the simple resultant of the work of each of these forces, or they may be set in opposition or not follow the simple compositional laws of vectorial addition. The proposition concerning the genesis of discharge and overflow of affects from the conflict of drive forces and restraining (structural) forces, as well as propositions concerning the origin and effects of signal affects, imply an action of forces according to other laws than those of simple vectorial composition.

The *structural point of view* demands that psychoanalytic explanation include propositions concerning abiding psychological configurations (structures). It assumes that there are psychological structures that are configurations of a slow rate of change and that these are hierarchically ordered. Mental processes are conceived of as taking place within, between, and by means of the organization of these structural configurations.

The *genetic point of view* demands that psychoanalytic explanation include propositions concerning psychological origin and development. It assumes that all psychological phenomena have such origins and developmental histories and that they originate in innate givens that mature according to an epigenetic plan. Earlier forms of a psychological phenomenon remain potentially active, although they may be superseded by later forms. At each point of psychological history, the totality of potentially active earlier forms codetermines all subsequent psychological phenomena.

Consequently, the psychoanalytic view of development postulates the gradual emergence of intrinsic maturational factors as innate givens that operate on a more or less preset timetable. These intrinsic factors are influenced by a complex and continuing interaction with experiential factors during the course of development. Development is thus the outcome of nature-and-nurture and not the result of either to the exclusion of the other. It is particularly important to emphasize that the experiential aspects of development are not simply stimulus inputs in the sense implied by the rather impersonal designation "average expectable environment" but, rather, are provided by the specific context of object relationships within which the developmental experience takes place. There is thus an interplay between maturational factors and developmental learning, such learning taking place within the context of object relationships provided by the child's significant caretakers.

Freud alluded to the relationship between the constitutional-maturational and environmental-experiential factors in his discussion of "complemental series." He observed in 1905:

> It is not easy to estimate the relative efficacy of the constitutional and accidental factors. In theory one is always inclined to overestimate the former; therapeutic practice emphasizes the importance of the latter. It should, however, on no account be forgotten that the relation between the two is a co-operative and not a mutually exclusive one. The constitutional factor must await experiences before it can make itself felt; the accidental factor must have a constitutional basis in order to come into operation. To cover the majority of cases we can picture what has been described as a "complemental series," in which the diminishing intensity of one factor is balanced by the increasing intensity of the other. . . . [7 *SE* 239–240]

Hartmann and Kris in 1945 added an important point by emphasizing that the genetic or developmental point of view did not concern itself simply with recovery of past events but, rather, with the causal sequencing of developmental effects at various levels of the developmental experience. They put it in the following terms:

> The genetic approach in psychoanalysis does not deal only with anamnestic data, nor does it intend to show only "how the past is contained in the present." Genetic propositions describe why, in past situations of conflict, a specific solution was adopted; why the one was retained and the other dropped, and what causal relation exists between these solutions and later developments. [1945:17]

There is a double emphasis in the psychoanalytic notion of development and in the genetic point of view that demands to be highlighted. From one point of view, the genetic hypothesis stresses the understanding of psychological processes as antecedent determinants, whereas from a second perspective the genetic point of view stresses the role of developmental transformations; that is, the influence of progressive and regressive processes on the changing organization of the psyche. The view in terms of antecedent determinants, for example, asserts the direct effect of the past on current mental functioning, a point that Freud had emphasized in his statement made during the period between 1893 and 1895 that "Hysterics suffer mainly from reminiscences" (2 SE 7). The role of antecedent determinants is also seen in the effect of infantile fantasies in determining later character and symptom formation. This view of antecedent determinants has clinical application in the understanding and interpretation of transference and in the use of genetic reconstruction.

The transformational view, however, places the emphasis on the consequences of sequential genetic transformations, whether progressive or regressive, as determinants of current psychic functioning and behavior. Although historical precursors have an inevitable influence on the course of such functioning, each phase in the developmental progression reflects a new organizational achievement that stands on its own without reference to specific antecedents. The genetic perspective within psychoanalysis embraces both genetic precursors as antecedent determinants and the capacity for genetic transformations as part of the ongoing process of the individual's life history that expresses the continuing operation of causal antecedents in current adaptations.

The developmental viewpoint within psychoanalysis provides a far-reaching schema for the organization of analytical data and for the generation of specific explanatory schemata. The analyst is concerned, therefore, not merely with establishing the current effects of antecedent contexts, circumstances, traumata, or affective fixations on the patient's current conflict and behavior, but also with seeking a broader understanding of those causal determinants, which may have brought about one set of behaviors or responses at an earlier stage of developmental interaction and may correspondingly operate in similar or in modified ways to generate current conflicts and behavioral difficulties. The developmental viewpoint, therefore, provides a complex lens or frame of reference through which it is possible to focus the interplay of important factors in the organization and functioning of the patient's personality. As such, it is capable of providing an integrative context for the understanding of the interaction of the rest of the metapsychological assumptions.

The *adaptive point of view* demands that psychoanalytic explanation include propositions concerning relationships to the environment. It assumes that there are psychological states of adaptiveness and processes of adaptation that apply at every point of psychological experience. Adaptive processes are autoplastic or alloplastic, or both, and operate to maintain, restore, or improve existing states of adaptiveness, which thereby ensure fitting in with the environment and survival. Human adaptation is not merely environmental but also social, applying both to the physical and human environments. Adaptational relationships are mutual in the sense that man and environment adapt to each other and, in the further sense, that human beings and their significant objects adapt to each other. Again, Rapaport comments:

> It is not yet possible to assess whether all these assumptions are necessary, and whether this set of assumptions is sufficient—when coupled with observational data—to yield the existing body of psychoanalytic propositions. Such an assessment could be achieved only by systematic study, by continuing to subject psychoanalytic propositions to an analysis which would strip away their empirical

content and establish whether or not their postulational (nonempirical) implications are accounted for by this set of assumptions. The future development of psychoanalysis as a systematic science may well depend on such continuing efforts to establish the assumptions on which psychoanalytic theory rests. [1967:809–810]

TEN

Ongoing Developments

Object Relations Theory

One of the currents in psychoanalysis, running its course of development, in a sense, parallel to the line of psychoanalytic ego psychology that has been traced in the preceding pages, is the approach to psychoanalysis through object relations theory. Only recently have the parallel and somewhat independent courses of theoretical development begun to converge. The development of classical psychoanalytic theory through the elaboration of a systematic ego psychology has led inexorably in the direction of a better understanding of the adaptive functions of the ego, particularly the close involvement between the ego and reality in its functioning and its development. One important dimension of the problem of reality in psychoanalytic theory is the whole question of object relations. The problem of integrating these two currents of analytic thinking remains a present theoretical concern within psychoanalysis.

Origins

The origins of the object relations view can best be traced from the contribution of Melanie Klein. Klein had originally trained with Karl Abraham in Berlin, and during the late 1920s and subsequent decades, she undertook extensive investigations of childhood pathologies in an attempt to document and refine some of Abraham's views about mental development and its pathological deviations. Klein's theorizing based itself primarily on the death instinct as the main theoretical prop of her metapsychology. Her major emphasis fell on the developmental vicissitudes of the superego. She extended this approach to the study of the fantasies and behaviors of severely disturbed children into a full-scale analysis of the internal psychic world and its development.

She saw the superego as an endopsychic organization that developed independently of biological influences and was determined entirely by the pattern of the child's relationship to the parents and the vicissitudes of the primary instincts. Klein's emphasis in the child's developmental experience fell on the processes of introjection and projection, derived from basic instinctual drives, and their interactions with the important and primary objects of the child's early experience. The emphasis on the relationship with objects and the delineation of the internal structuring of the child's inner fantasy world in terms of the vicissitudes of introjects provided the basis and the rudimentary content for an object relations view of development.

Thus Klein's "inner world" was peopled by internal objects that were either good or bad and with whom the individual was involved in intrapsychic interactions and struggles that were in many ways as real as those carried on with the real objects outside the person. In fact, Klein saw external object relations as derived from and influenced by projective content derived from the internal object relations. Klein has been generously criticized for her almost blind interpretation of all forms of aggressive or destructive intent as manifestations of the death instinct, for her failure to distinguish among the various kinds of intrapsychic content (lumping object representations, self-representations, internal objects, fantasies, and psychic structures of various kinds together indiscriminately and treating them in a unitary fashion), for her tendency to substitute theoretical inferences for observations and, finally, for her marked tendency to predate the emergence of intrapsychic organizations that are generally thought by other theorists to be achieved only in later developmental stages, for example, locating the origin of the superego in the first year of life.

In any case, Klein's observations and formulations had a tremendous impact, particularly in bringing into prominence the role of aggression in pathological development, in making theorists of development much more aware of the early developmental precursors of later structural entities, and particularly in providing the basic rudiments and foundations for an emergent theory of object relations. Although Klein's emphasis was primarily on the world of internal objects rather than on the ego, and more strongly on the role of instincts in the intrapsychic dynamics rather than on the objects themselves, subsequent theorists have followed her lead and have shifted the emphasis from the instinctual basis, which was more classically Freudian, to an emphasis on the objects and the external environment.

Ego and Objects

Beginning in about 1931, Ronald Fairbairn shifted the emphasis in his thinking specifically to the problems of ego analysis. Fairbairn's contribution was to bring personal object relations into the center of the theory. Following Klein's analysis of the internalized psychic object, Fairbairn proposed a radical ego analysis. Whereas the ego in Freudian theory had been regarded as a superficial modification of the id, developed specifically for the purpose of impulse control and adaptation to the demands of reality, Fairbairn conceived of the ego as the core phenomenon of the psyche. Rather than an organization of functions, he conceived of it more specifically as real self; that is, the dynamic center or core of the personality. Instead of basing his theory on the instinctual drives as the basic concept, Fairbairn shifted the emphasis to the ego and saw everything in human psychology as specifically an effect of ego-functioning.

With this reorientation, there came a reformulation of the instinctual perspective. The libido or the instincts in general, rather than mechanisms for energic discharge, were regarded as essentially object-seeking. Erotogenic zones were not the primary determinants of libidinal aims but, rather, channels that mediated the primary relationships with objects, particularly with relationships with objects that had been internalized during early life under the pressure of deprivation and frustration. Ego development itself was characterized by a process whereby an original state of infantile dependence, based on a symbiotic union with the maternal object, was abandoned in favor of a state of adult or mature dependence that was based on differentiation between self and object. Thus, Fairbairn conceptualized the developmental process as the vicissitudes of objects, rather than the vicissitudes of instincts.

The basis for much of Fairbairn's theorizing was his experience with schizoid patients. He contrasted the basic dilemma of the schizoid with that of neurotic patients on whom classical psychoanalytic theory was based. He saw that the schizoid was not primarily concerned with control of threatening impulses toward significant objects, but that the issue for this patient was essentially a question of having an ego capable of forming object relations at all. The relationship to objects presented a difficulty, not because of dangerous impulses arising in connection with them, but because the ego was weak, undeveloped, infantile, and fragile. In the struggle to overcome this inner weakness, the schizoid's impulses became antisocial.

The schizoid's problem is, at bottom, a question of an infantile ego unable to cope with the world of objects. Thus, in one's growing emotional life, the schizoid is split by the inconsistency in primary objects and becomes a victim of the loss of internal unity and of personal radical helplessness. The internalized objects are split into good and bad objects, which cannot be amalgamated. Parallel to the split in objects, there is within the ego itself a radical split that calls for a different conception of intrapsychic structure than that provided by the classical psychoanalytic model.

Schizoid individuals experience themselves as empty, meaningless, worthless, lonely, isolated, and craving for close contact with objects for the sake of preserving a sense of security. Such psychodynamic security can be achieved only by the adequate growth of the ego, fostered and initiated by what Winnicott calls "good-enough mothering." Fairbairn points out that the model for splitting of the ego was provided by Freud in his analysis of the superego, which he described initially as a "differentiating grade of the ego." Whereas Freud's analysis of splitting was based on the phenomenon of depression and unconscious guilt, the object relations approach bases its analysis of splitting on the schizoid problem.

Thus, object relations theory in its bare essentials contains a number of basic points that differentiate it from classical theory. First, the ego is conceived of as whole or total at birth, becoming split or losing inner unity as a result of early bad experiences in object relationships, particularly in relation to the mothering object. This point is quite opposite to the classical theory, according to which the ego begins as undifferentiated and unintegrated and only achieves unity through the course of development. Second, the libido is regarded as a primary life drive of the psyche, the energic source of the ego's search for the relatedness with good objects, which makes ego growth possible. Third, aggression is regarded as a natural defensive reaction to the frustration of the libidinal drive, rather than specifically as an independent instinct. Fourth, the structural ego pattern that emerges when the pristine ego unity is lost involves a pattern of ego splitting and the formation of internal ego-object relations.

The shift in emphasis toward the primacy of the external environment and the influence of objects on the course of development has established a definite trend in psychoanalytic thinking and has been advanced primarily in the work of British theorists, among whom one can point particularly to the work of Michael Balint and Donald Winnicott. Winnicott particularly has emphasized the importance of early interactions between mother and child as determining factors in the laying down of important components of ego development. Currently, there is ample room for overlap in the approaches and formulations of both the object relations theorists and the more classical psychoanalytic ego theorists.

Both Balint and Winnicott, in company with other object relations theorists, were concerned with levels of early developmental failure that are essentially preoedipal, that are manifested in forms of personality disorder that are more primitive and more difficult to treat than the usual neurotic disorders, and that do not fit well with the classical psychoanalytic structural theory with its basic focus on issues of intrapsychic conflict.

Balint envisioned several layers of psychological functioning in analysis. The first is the familiar genital level, centering on triadic relationships and concerned specifically with intrapsychic conflicts. These conflicts and quality of relationships are the usual material of an analysis and can be treated by adult language. There is, however, a second, deeper level at which the conventional meaning of words no longer has the same impact and at which interpretations are no longer perceived as meaningful by the patient. This is the level of preverbal experience. Balint recognized that at this level of preverbal experience an attempt to address or describe the child's experience in adult language is bound to fail. Problems arise in analysis when efforts are made to interpret events from this preverbal level in adult terms.

Balint distinguished between phases of regression that he described as benign and malignant. The benign regression is more or less an extension of the basic notion of the analytic regression to a level of primitive relationship with the primary objects. Such a regression is gradual, tempered, and modulated according to the patient's capacity to tolerate and productively integrate the resulting anxiety. During this regression, the analyst's empathic responsiveness and recognition make it possible for the patient to withstand this unstructured experience and to keep the anxiety within manageable limits. At the level of the basic fault, the lost infantile objects can be mourned, and the quality of the relationship with them is open to reworking so that the patient's basic assumptions that govern the interaction with the object world can be reformed.

During phases of the benign regression to this preverbal and pregenital level of object relationship in the analysis, the analyst can usually provide an empathic acceptance and recognition, rather than verbalized interpretations, along with a patient tolerance of this level of the patient's unstructured experience, without anxiety or the need to escape or the need to subvert this level of experience through interpretation. Balint felt that the dynamics at this level are more primitive than can be adequately expressed as conflict because they derive from the basic form of dual relationship involved in the early mother-child interaction. He referred to this level of impairment in object relations as the "basic fault."

In contrast, malignant regression tends to be precipitous and extreme; the ego is prematurely overwhelmed by traumatic and unmanageable anxiety. This anxiety prevents any effective reworking of fundamental disturbances in object relationships, re-creating and reinforcing the basic fault, rather than creating the conditions for its therapeutic revision.

At an even deeper level, beyond the reach of analytic resources, there lies the area of creativity; that is, an idiosyncratic, uncommunicable, and objectless area that lies beyond conventional expression.

Regression to the level of the basic fault is a quite different and distinct phenomenon than the more usual oedipal regressions experienced in the analysis of adult neurotics. In the oedipal regression the aim is gratification of infantile instinctual wishes. Regression to the level of the basic fault, however, seeks a basic recognition by the therapist, as well as protective support and consent to express the inner core of creativity that lies at the heart of the patient's being and accounts for the capacity to become ill or well. Balint uses the notion of primary love at this deepest level to describe the withdrawal of libido from the frustrating object in an attempt to reestablish a certain inner harmony in which it becomes possible to recover the conditions of early care and tranquillity. He refers to a "harmonious interpenetrating mix-up" to describe the early, almost undifferentiated interaction of the infant and environment. The analogy is that of breathing air; the organism cannot exist without air, so air and the organism are seemingly inseparable, but to cut off the supply of air reveals both the organism's need of it and the distinction between air and the organism. In terms of primary love, then, the patient seeks a basic form of recognition from the analyst, as from the significant objects in the patient's life.

Winnicott also was concerned with the earliest phase of the mother-child relationship and the importance of what he described as "good-enough mothering" for the child's personality development. The course of development involves a movement from an early stage of total or absolute dependence, analogous to Mahler's symbiotic phase, toward a more adult phase of relative independence. As he saw it, the inherited native potential for growth was strongly influenced by the quality of maternal care. This potential for development is affected even from the moment of conception. Even before birth, the child becomes invested by a strong narcissistic cathexis that allows the mother to identify with the child and to become empathically attuned to the child's inner needs, as if the child were—and indeed is—an extension of her own self. Winnicott calls this early prenatal involvement of mother and child-in-the-womb a "primary maternal preoccupation." This sets the stage for the development of a holding relationship, in which the mother becomes sensitively attuned to the infant's needs and sensitivities and is both physically and emotionally responsive to them, thus providing a physical, physiological, and emotional ambiance, protection, and security for the absolutely dependent infant.

As the infant moves from this early stage of absolute dependence toward a more relative dependence, awareness of personal needs and of the existence of the mother as a caretaking object grows. The optimal relationship at this stage involves a continuation of the protective holding, along with an optimal titration of gratification and frustration. As a result of this optimally attuned relationship between the patterning of infantile drives and initiatives and their harmonious fitting in with maternal sensitivities and responsiveness, there is a developing sense of reliable expectation that the infant's needs will be satisfied without the threat of excessive withdrawal of the mothering object and without the threatening, overwhelming, and short-circuiting of the infant's initiatives as a result of excessive maternal impingements.

In the course of normal development, this allows for the emergence of a certain omnipotence from which the child gradually retreats with the experiences of tolerable degrees of frustration and separateness of the maternal object. Although the mother continues her holding at this phase, she must yet allow enough separation between herself and the developing infant to permit the expression of the baby's needs and initiatives that form the rudiments of the emerging sense of self. If she is too distant, too unresponsive, or not sufficiently present, anxiety arises and is accompanied by the fading of the infant's internal representations of her.

The transition from a phase of absolute dependence to one of relative dependence represents a crucial development in the capacity for object relations. It is accompanied by a critical transition from total subjectivity to the capacity for objectivity in the perception of and relation to objects. The transition from subjectivity to objectivity is accomplished by the development of Winnicott's transitional phenomenon, expressed in the first instance in the emergence of transitional objects. These objects are the child's first object possessions that are perceived as separate from the emerging self—the first "not me" possessions. From the study of infant behavior, Winnicott argued that the object is a substitute for the maternal breast, the first and most significant object in the environment to which the infant relates. The transitional object exists in an intermediate realm contributed to both by the external reality of the object (the mother's breast) and by the child's own subjectivity. This intermediate realm is at once both subjective and objective without being exclusively either.

Winnicott refers to this realm as the realm of illusion, an intermediate area of experience that embraces both inner and external reality and may be retained in areas of adult functioning having to do with such imaginative capacities as creativity, religious experience, and art. In its primitive form, however, the transitional object commonly experienced in childhood development may take the form of a particular object, a blanket, a pillow, or a favorite toy or teddy bear to which the child becomes intensely attached and from which it cannot be separated without the stirring up of severe anxiety and distress. Attachment to this object is an immediate displacement from the figure of the mother and represents an important developmental step, insofar as it allows the child to tolerate increasing degrees of separation from the mother, using the transitional object as a substitute.

The mother participates in this intermediate transitional realm of illusion by her responsiveness to the infant's need to continually create her as a good mother. In her sensitivity and responsiveness, she functions as a good-enough mother. However, her failure to provide such adequate mothering, either by excessive withdrawal or by excessive intrusion and control, may result in the emergence of a false self in the child based on compliance with the demands of the external environment, a condition that reflects a developmental failure and results in a variety of often severe character pathologies.

When such patients are seen as adults, they are neither neurotic nor psychotic, but seem to relate to the world through a compliant shell that is not quite real to them or to the analyst. They are mistrustful without being specifically paranoid, they appear withdrawn and disengaged and seem able to relate only by means of the protective shell, which seems apparently obsessive and compliant but which separates and isolates them from meaningful contacts with their fellows, even as it provides their only basis for relationship. These disturbed personality types reflect a basic impairment in very early object relations, particularly in the mutuality and responsiveness of the very early mother-child interaction.

Infants who develop in the direction of a false self mode have not experienced the security and mutual satisfaction of such a relationship. Such mothers are empathically out of contact with the child and react largely on the basis of their own inner fantasies, narcissistic needs, or neurotic conflicts. The child's survival depends on the capacity to adapt to this pattern of the mother's response, which is so grossly out of phase with the child's needs. This establishes a pattern of gradual training in compliance with whatever the mother is capable of offering, rather than the seeking out and finding of what is needed and wanted. Consequently, the child's needs, instinctual impulses, wishes and initiatives, instead of becoming a meaningful guide to satisfying growth experiences and the enlarging capacities to interact meaningfully with objects, become from the very beginning a threat to the harmony of the relationship with the mother, who remains unresponsive to any feedback from the child.

Winnicott's attempts to formulate principles of treatment for such basically impaired patients build on the model of good-enough mothering. This called for a capacity for holding, for empathic responsiveness, and for a capacity for creatively playful exchange that allows the patient's capacities for growth to emerge and flourish, permitting the expansion of the patient's authentic sense of self, which remains hidden behind the external facade of the false-self compliance.

Although many contemporary analysts would argue that Freud's instinct theory can in no way be conceived as excluding the importance of objects and the significance of the influence of objects as internal psychic development, there are specific problems that remain to be resolved. Particular theoretical issues that reveal some divergence in these approaches have to do specifically with the character of the ego. In the object relations approach, the ego seems to expand to encompass the whole of the internal psychic structure. Moreover, it is conceived of as a unitary structure in the beginning of the child's experience with objects. These propositions stand in direct opposition to the classical notion of the ego as a substructural organization within the psychic apparatus. It also stands in opposition to the basic Freudian notion of the infant beginning life in a state of objectless primary narcissism and developing gradually in the direction of object libido and object attachment. The last critical area of divergence between these theories is between the concept of ego as an organization of functions (functional ego) in the classical approach and the concept of ego as more closely identified with the objectively experienced real self (personal ego) in the object relations approach.

Psychology of the Self

Over the last score and more of years, the concept of the self has been emerging with increasing emphasis and definition as a central notion in the deepening psychoanalytic understanding of the organization and functioning of the human psyche. Although the concepts regarding the understanding of the self are still very much in flux, and the place of the notion of the self in psychoanalytic theory remains tentative and uncertain, the issues addressed by the psychology of the self seem to be of sufficient significance and to have gained a more or less permanent place in psychoanalytic thinking, so that a consideration of these issues is warranted in this presentation.

The issues to which a self-psychology addresses itself are by no means new to psychoanalysis. Part of the problem stems from the ambiguity in Freud's use of the term *ich*, standing ambiguously both for the ego as part of the mental apparatus, a structural agency, and for the more experiential subjective and personal sense of self. The decision of the editors of the English *Standard Edition* to translate *ich* by the term "ego" tended to shift the meaning of the term toward the more impersonal structural sense of agency and away from the more subjective experiential implications. There are passages where it is quite clear that Freud uses the German term *selbst* as synonymous with the term *ich*, referring to the subjectively experienced self, the person as such.

This unresolved ambiguity and the progressive shift in implications of the term "ego" have left a certain vacuum in psychoanalytic metapsychology. This deficit has been attacked by a number of thinkers as reflecting a lack of personal ego or a sense of self-as-agent in psychoanalytic theory.

Partly in an attempt to deal with this issue, the notion of the self has been focused by various analytic thinkers in a variety of contexts. Adler, for example, connected the notion of the self with the individual's style of life, which referred to the unique and individual personality that reflected the individual's creative capacity to compensate for feelings of inferiority. For Jung, the self was a primordial image or archetype, expressing the need for unity and wholeness and reflecting the individual's individuation and life goals that gave existence meaning and purpose. Horney also stressed the notions of unity and purpose, as well as the capacity to develop one's own authentic goals and to become an active instrument in leading one's own life. As she saw it, the root of neurosis lay in the alienation of the idealized self from the real self, the ideal self standing for the individual's personal goals and ideals. Sullivan also speaks of a self-dynamism or a self-system, the purpose of which is the fulfillment of needs and the preservation and maintenance of emotional security. Consistent with his interpersonal view, the self in Sullivan's theory primarily reflects the vicissitudes of interpersonal relationships. Finally, Kohut's more recent focus on the self has been a major stimulus of the renewed interest.

The Psychology of Character

The development of the concept of character in psychoanalysis has drawn increasingly closer to the issues that are latent in a psychology of the self. Character has come to stand for a unique combination of the components of the individual's psychic organization that reflects the basic elements of that person's personality organization and style. The implications of the concept of character, then, lie much closer to the framework of the personality functioning as a whole, rather than to specific psychic agencies.

Historical Development

The concept of character can vary widely in meaning, depending on whether it is used in a moralistic, literary, sociological, or general sense. The application of the concept in psychoanalysis has remained restrictive despite the fact that theoretical propositions that have been advanced concerning the meaning of character have undergone an evolution that parallels the evolution in psychoanalytic theory, particularly in the theory of the ego. During the period when Freud was developing his instinct theory, he noted the relationship between certain character traits and particular psychosexual components. For example, he recognized that obstinacy, orderliness, and parsimoniousness were associated with anality. He noted that ambition was related to urethral eroticism and that generosity was related to orality. He concluded, in his paper on "Character and Anal Eroticism," that permanent character traits represented "unchanged prolongations of the original instincts, or sublimation of those instincts, or reaction-formations against them" (9 *SE* 175).

In 1913, Freud made an important distinction between neurotic symptoms and character traits: neurotic symptoms come into being as a result of the failure of repression, the return of the repressed; charac-

ter traits owe their existence to the success of repression or, more accurately, of the defense system, which achieves its aim through a persistent pattern of reaction formation and sublimation. Later, in 1923, with
increased understanding of the phenomenon of identification and the
formulation of the ego as a coherent system of functions, the relationship of character to ego development came into sharper focus. At this
point, Freud observed that the replacement of object attachment by
identification (introjection), which set up the lost object inside the
ego, also made a significant contribution to character formation. A
decade later, in 1932, Freud emphasized the particular importance of
identification (introjection) with the parents for the construction of
character, particularly with reference to superego formation.

Several of Freud's disciples made important contributions to the
concept of character during this period. A major share of Karl Abraham's efforts were devoted to the investigation and elucidation of
the relationship between oral, anal, and genital eroticism and various
character traits. Wilhelm Reich made an important contribution to
the psychoanalytic understanding of character when he described the
intimate relationship between resistance in treatment and character
traits of the patient's personality. Reich's observation that resistance
typically appeared in the form of these specific traits anticipated Anna
Freud's later formulation concerning the relationship between resistances and typical ego defenses.

The development of psychoanalytic ego psychology has led to an
increasing tendency to include character and character traits among
the properties of the ego, superego, and ego-ideal. It should be noted,
however, that character is not synonymous with any of these properties. Concomitantly, the emphasis has been extended from an interest
in specific character traits to a consideration of character and its formation in general. Psychoanalysis has come to regard character as the
pattern of adaptation to instinctual and environmental forces, which
is typical or habitual for a given individual. The character of a person
is distinguished from the ego by virtue of the fact that it refers largely
to directly observable behavior and styles of defense, as well as of acting, thinking, and feeling. The clinical value of the concept of character has been recognized by psychiatrists and psychoanalysts and has
become a meeting ground for the two disciplines.

Evolution of Character

The formation of character and character traits results from the interplay of multiple factors. Innate biological predisposition plays a role in character formation in both its instinctual and ego fundaments. The interactions of id forces with early ego defenses and with environmental influences, particularly the parents, constitutes the major determinants in the development of character. Various early identifications and imitations of objects leave their lasting stamp on character formation.

The degree to which the ego has developed a capacity to tolerate delay in drive discharge and to neutralize instinctual energies, as a result of early identifications and defense formation, determines the later emergence of such character traits as impulsiveness. Finally, a number of authors have stressed the particularly close association between character traits and the development of the ego-ideal. The development of the ego-ideal must be understood in the context of the developmental vicissitudes of narcissism. It is in this respect that the psychoanalytic concept of character begins to parallel the more common use of the term "character" in a somewhat moral sense. The exaggerated development of certain character traits at the expense of others may lead to character disorders in later life. At other times, such distortions in the development of character traits produce a vulnerability in personality organization or a predisposition to psychotic decompensation.

Identity

A significant contribution in the evolution toward a more articulated notion of the self was provided in Erik Erikson's formulations of the notions of identity and identity formation. The concepts have remained somewhat global in their implications and have not as yet attained any definitive position in psychoanalytic theory. The concept of identity undoubtedly retains close links with both the notion of the ego and with the notion of the self, but the specific relationships have yet to be defined and depend in part on the determination of the theoretical links between the notion of the self and the components of the structural theory, particularly id, ego, and superego. Erikson's own use of the term seems to vary between giving it specific reference to the ego and referring it more globally to the total personality organization as such. In any case, the focusing of the notion of identity raises questions about its integration with the concept of the self. One of the primary issues in the psychoanalytic theory of the self has to do not only with its relationship to aspects of the tripartite structural theory but also with its connection with the vicissitudes of narcissistic development. In this sense the notion of identity can be seen as providing an important bridge between the psychology of character and the psychology of the self.

In Erikson's terms, then, the notion of identity seems to refer to a complex set of implications, including a conscious sense of individual identity or subjective self-experience, an unconscious striving for continuity of personal character, the effects of ego synthesis, and finally, a sense of inner solidarity with the ideals and identity of a social group. The achievement of identity is assigned to the adolescent period; the developmental tasks of adolescence are completed when the individual is able to subordinate childhood identifications and to fashion them into a new synthesis, representing the creative achievement of an individual sense of identity and its associated life commitments. The psychosocial moratorium provided by late latency and adolescence provides the opportunity for testing out various identifications and social roles, which allows the emerging young adult to gain an assured sense of inner psychic continuity and external social acknowledgment that affords bridging the gap between the childhood being lost and the adulthood about to be accomplished. As Erikson himself observes,

> *Identity formation,* finally, begins where the usefulness of identification ends. It arises from the selective repudiation and mutual assimilation of childhood identifications, and their absorption in a new configuration, which in turn, is dependent on the process by which a *society* (often through subsocieties) *identifies the young individual,* recognizing him as somebody who had to become the way he is, and who, being the way he is, is taken for granted. [1959:113]

Thus, Erikson's notion of identity seems to provide a term to express the sense of continuity and coherence of the organization of the self, and at the same time it articulates certain aspects of the engagement of the self with its objects and with its shaping social environment. Identity, then, can be regarded as referring to a specific aspect of the self-organization and functioning. In this light, it can be seen as an effort to deal with the latent ambiguity in psychoanalytic thinking regarding the place of the subjectively experienced personal sense of self and, at the same time, as an attempt to articulate the role of the self vis-à-vis the object world.

Evolving Concepts of the Self

The direct line of development of the notion of the self in psychoanalysis can probably be best traced back to the effort of Hartmann to clarify the ambiguity latent in Freud's use of the term *ich*. Hartmann distinguished ego from the self by assigning the respective terms to different frames of explanatory reference. The ego referred to the specific intrapsychic agency whose frame of reference and action was within the intrapsychic structure and in relationship to the other tripartite entities, namely, superego and id. The self, in contrast, had its proper frame of reference in relationship to the notion of object. Thus formulated, the notion of the self came to be regarded as roughly equivalent to the concept of the person.

In an effort to clarify the theoretical implications of the self, early thinkers, following Hartmann's lead, came to define the term in representational terms; that is, as referring to the self-representation, which was then regarded as a subordinate function of the ego. Another point of view, however, would see the self as a structural organization, either envisioned as a fourth focus of organization in addition to the tripartite entities or as a supraordinate organization that includes the tripartite structures and perhaps additional structural aspects.

Part of the difficulty is that the notion of the self can be looked at from a variety of perspectives. The self can be seen as agent, or as object, or even in locational terms, with respect to questions of what is inside or outside of the mind or the psychic structure and what it might mean for parts of the self to be internalized or externalized. The representational view of the self seems to lend itself most clearly to a view of the self as object; that is, as what can be cognitively and experientially grasped of the self as an object of inner experience. Such an experienced object must have representational qualities to be cognitively relevant. By the same token, the structural perspective seems to be most congruent with the view of the self as agent, as a source of psychic integration and activity, and as synonymous with the originating source of personal action and awareness. The structural aspect of the self as agent comes closest to satisfying the demand for a "personal ego" in the theory.

The theory of the self remains at this juncture uncertain and very much in flux. However the ultimate conceptualization may be resolved, it seems apparent that the psychology of the self will continue to gain a permanent place in psychoanalytic thinking and theory. It is possible to specify some of the theoretical gains of the emerging role of the self-concept in the theory:

1. The self as a theoretical construct provides a focus for formulating and understanding the complex integrations of functional processes that involve combinations of functions of the respective component agencies. This would have specific application to such complex activities as affects, in which all of the psychic systems seem to be in one way or other represented; complex superego integrations reflected in such formations as value systems; and other complex interactions of psychic systems that involve fantasy production, drive-motor integration, or cognitive-affective processes. There is room here for considerable reworking and refocusing of traditional psychoanalytic ways of looking at and understanding psychic phenomena in terms of the self as a referent system.
2. The self-concept provides a more specific and less ambiguous frame of reference for the articulation of self-object interrelationships and interactions, including the complex areas of object relations and internalizations.
3. The emergence of a self-concept provides a locus in the theory for articulating the experience of the personal self, either as grasped introspectively and reflectively or experienced as the originating source of personal activity. This would provide a place within the theory for an account of subjectivity and subjective meaning.

This approach raises an important metapsychological issue; namely, the relationship between the experienced organization of the self and the tripartite entities. The organization of the self and the organization of structural tripartite entities cannot be simply identified. The self-organization operates at a different level of psychic organization than do the structural entities; moreover, the structural entities in the strict theoretical sense are understood to be organizations of specific functions. This concept applies not only to the ego as such but also to the superego and the id. Although the theory at various points attributes more or less personalized, anthropomorphized metaphors to the operation of these structures, their strict theoretical intelligibility is nonetheless given in terms of the organization of specific functions attributed to the respective structures.

A defect in the structural theory and a source of considerable confusion in psychoanalytic thinking is that it has difficulty integrating and accounting for complex experiential states. One of the major difficulties in the structural concept is that it leaves no room for the experience of one's own self as an integrated and relatively autonomous self-originating focus of action. If the realm of subjective experience can be specifically related to the cognition of and organization of the self, then there is room for a subjective experience of self as an active and organizing principle within the intrapsychic apparatus.

ELEVEN

Classical Psychoanalytic Treatment

CERTAIN ASPECTS of the therapeutic technique that Freud developed and that were later expanded by his followers bear a close relationship with the aspects of psychoanalytic theory discussed in this essay. One of the distinctive aspects of the psychoanalytic approach to treatment in general is its consistent attempt to integrate therapeutic usages and approaches with the understanding of psychic functioning available from psychoanalytic theory. In its origins and in its special application, psychoanalysis is uniquely a theory of therapy.

Before turning to a discussion of some aspects of the analytic treatment process, it is well to approach the problem from the vantage point from which it all begins, namely, diagnosis. In any systematic approach to the treatment of emotional illness, diagnosis must hold a central place because the decisions regarding the appropriate form of treatment depend on the accuracy and precision of the diagnostic process. This remains generally as true for psychoanalytic treatment as for any psychiatric or medical intervention.

It must be appreciated, however, that the diagnostic process represents an attempt to impose categories on an underlying continuum of infinitely variable forms of illness. Consequently, no diagnostic system is definitive, and no diagnostic system answers to all of the decisional needs that relate to the treatment process. One important result of this state of affairs is that multiple diagnostic schemata have been evolved throughout the history of psychiatry. The kind of schema developed depends to a very large extent on the purposes for which it is formulated and the objectives to which it is directed. Thus, the spectrum of psychiatric illnesses can be grouped and categorized in different ways depending on the purposes and objectives of that set of categories.

To the extent that the objectives and purposes of psychoanalytic treatment are congruent with and overlap the objectives of general psychiatry, one would expect that a psychoanalytic diagnostic rationale would coincide with the psychiatric. A cursory glance through the following forms of psychopathology described from a psychoanalytic perspective would suggest that there is a considerable degree of overlap with general psychiatric categories, as exemplified in the *Diagnostic and Statistical Manual of Mental Disorders* (DSM).

The alert reader, however, will also notice that there are significant differences. Consequently, it should be emphasized that the basis for psychoanalytic diagnosis differs from that of a more general psychiatric approach. That approach can be described as descriptive, observational, and extrinsic. The analytic approach, in contrast, has emphasized the patient's inner experience, particularly the quality of the patient's inner conflicts and related fantasies, as an important component of the diagnostic evaluation. As the psychoanalytic perspective has evolved, however, analytic diagnosis has extended its reach into such pertinent areas as assessment of the degree of autonomy of ego functions and their susceptibility to regression, as well as the quality, both historically and contemporaneously, of the patient's object relationships—including the therapeutic relationship, specifically in the evaluation of the transference and other dimensions of the complex relationship that arises between analyst and patient.

Psychoanalytic Psychopathology

Psychoanalytic theories concerning mental disorders have undergone extensive expansion and modification since Freud discovered the free association method of investigation. These theories have retained their emphasis on the investigation of etiological factors, rather than in the mere description of symptoms. By 1906, Freud had succeeded in understanding the psychological processes underlying many mental disorders to a degree sufficient to permit him to classify them on the basis of psychopathology. At that point of his investigation, Freud's theory contained most of the major elements of present-day psychoanalytic concepts of psychopathology. He had advanced his initial hypotheses concerning the psychological mechanisms of the neuroses, character disorders, perversions, and psychoses.

Theory of Neurosis

The theory of neurosis in its traditional sense as referring to hysteria, obsessional neuroses, and phobias is central to the psychoanalytic concept of psychopathology. Neuroses develop under the following conditions: (1) There is an inner conflict between drives and fear that prevents drive discharge. (2) Sexual drives are involved in these conflicts. (3) Conflict has not been worked through to a realistic solution. Instead, the drives that seek discharge have been expelled from consciousness through repression or another defense mechanism. (4) Repression merely succeeded in rendering the drives unconscious; it did not deprive them of their power and make them innocuous. Consequently, the repressed tendencies have fought their way back to consciousness, now disguised as neurotic symptoms. (5) An inner conflict will lead to neurosis in adolescence or adulthood only if a neurosis, or a rudimentary neurosis based on the same type of conflict, existed in early childhood.

Character Disorders

In the section on the concept of psychoanalytic character in chapter 10, it was noted that the psychoanalytic sense of character refers to the individual's habitual mode of bringing into harmony the tasks presented by internal demands and the external world. When and how the individual acquires the qualities that make it possible to adjust, first to the demands of instinctual drives and of external reality and later to the demands of the superego, and how this adjustment is accomplished in varying degrees and styles of the functioning and adaptability of the ego could be the subject of a separate treatise. The description of pathological character types can be complex and confusing because personality types are rarely found in pure or discrete forms without considerable overlap with other character types.

Contemporary psychoanalysis is taken up with the diagnosis and treatment of character types more extensively than with any other aspect of psychopathology. It is quite frequently the case, when patients present with symptomatic complaints, that early in the treatment process symptomatic complaints are relieved but that, as treatment progresses, increasingly the problems of the underlying character structure become the focus of analytic treatment. Thus, there is a trend, often detectable in the course of therapy, from a focus on the issues of symptom formation to a focus on the problems of internal character structure, along with its concomitant issues of object relations. More prominently than in any other area of their disability, the character disorders reveal their malfunctioning in the area of object relationships.

A particular character pattern or type becomes pathological when its manifestations are exaggerated to the point that behavior destructive to the individual or to others is the result or when the functioning of the person becomes so disturbed or restricted that it becomes a source of distress to the person or to others. Characterological traits tend to be nearly lifelong and are usually deeply embedded in the organization of the individual's personality. The character types are usually classified according to associated symptomatic expression. Character disorders are also known as personality disorders.

The most useful division of character pathology has been provided by Kernberg in 1970. He includes the hysterical characters, obsessive-compulsive characters, and depressive-masochistic characters in his highest level of character pathology. "At the higher level," he states, "the patient has a relatively well-integrated but severe and punitive superego. . . . The patient's ego at this level is somewhat limited and constricted by its excessive use of neurotic defense mechanisms, but the patient's overall social adaptation is not seriously impaired" (1970:805).

At the intermediate level of character pathology, Kernberg emphasizes the defective integration of the superego, which is able to tolerate contradictory demands between sadistic, prohibitive superego nuclei, on the one hand, and rather primitive, magical, and somewhat idealizing nuclei, on the other. Kernberg goes on to say: "At the same time, the patient shows some dissociative trends, some defensive splitting of the ego in limited areas (that is, mutual dissociation of contradictory ego states), and projection and denial. Pregenital, especially oral, conflicts come to the fore, although the genital level of libidinal development has been reached" (1970:807).

Under this group Kernberg includes the oral types of character pathology, including passive-aggressive personalities, sadomasochistic personalities, some infantile personalities, and some narcissistic personalities.

At the lower level of character pathology, structural deficits and their developmental consequences are even more severe. "At the lower level," Kernberg writes, "the patient's superego integration is minimal and his propensity for projection of primitive, sadistic superego nuclei is maximal. . . . The synthetic function of the patient's ego is seriously impaired, and he uses primitive dissociation or splitting as the central defensive operation of the ego instead of repression . . ." (1970: 807, 808).

Included in this lowest bracket of character pathologies are the infantile personalities, many narcissistic personalities, antisocial personalities, the more chaotic impulse-ridden characters, the "as-if" characters, other patients with multiple sexual deviations in combination with drug addiction or alcoholism, and pathological object relationships, as well as other forms of schizoid and paranoid personality.

Narcissistic Character

Narcissistic characters present a pathological picture characterized by an excessive degree of self-reference in interaction with others, an excessive need to be loved and admired by others, and apparently contradictory attitudes of an inflated concept of themselves and an inordinate need for tribute and admiration from others. They often tend to idealize those from whom they expect narcissistic rewards, and conversely, they depreciate, devalue, and treat with contempt those from whom they cannot expect such rewards.

They experience little empathy for others. Their relationships with other people are often exploitative and manipulative. They seem to feel they have the right to control and possess others and to exploit them without guilt. Behind a facade that is often charming and engaging, there is a coldness and a ruthlessness that one senses rather than sees.

Although their need for admiration often makes them appear to be dependent, they characteristically have a deep distrust of others; yet envy is a strong characteristic of the narcissistic character.

Some of these patients present strong conscious feelings of inadequacy and inferiority that may at times alternate with feelings of importance, specialness, and omnipotent fantasies. Such extreme contradictions of self-concept are often the first clinical manifestations of the level of pathology and structural impairment of ego and superego hidden beneath a veneer of smooth and effective social functioning.

The narcissistic character disorders, however, differ markedly from the borderline or psychotic states in that these patients have attained a cohesive and organized self, and they are not threatened by the possibility of an irreversible decompensation of the organization of the self.

At the lowest level of character organization, the predominant forms are the schizoid personality and the borderline personality. In both of these personality configurations, the level of conflict and developmental fixation tends to be at a relatively primitive object relations type. The underlying conflicts for both personality types tend to be similar, but the pathological organization of defenses tends to follow different lines. The schizoid personality tends to follow a more obessional pattern of defense; the schizoid may be regarded as a more primitive and genetically earlier form of obsessional pathology. Consequently, many schizoid personalities tend to use obsessional defenses and often present clinically as obsessive-compulsive personalities. Borderline patients tend to follow a hysterical form of defensive organization and may be regarded as a more primitive form of hysterical pathology. Consequently, many borderline patients will present with hysterical features, except that these manifestations are more poorly organized and chaotic and more readily susceptible to regression.

Schizoid Character

The patient complains of feeling cut off, of being isolated and out of touch, of feeling apart or estranged from surrounding people and things, of things being somehow unreal, of diminishing interest in things and events, or of feeling life is futile and meaningless. Patients often call this state of mind "depression," but it lacks the inner sense of anger and guilt that is often easily discovered in depression. In depression it is often a struggle for the patient not to turn aggression outward into overt angry and destructive behavior. Depression is thus essentially object related. The schizoid character, however, has renounced objects.

The attitude to the outside world is one of noninvolvement and mere observation-at-a-distance without any feeling. The schizoid's major defense against anxiety is to keep emotionally out of reach, inaccessible, and isolated. The schizoid condition, then, consists of an attempt to cancel external object relations and to live in a detached and withdrawn manner.

The schizoid character is not far removed from the narcissistic character disorder. They often overlap considerably in their clinical description and in their underlying psychodynamics. The schizoid pathology often shows markedly narcissistic characteristics. The cold and isolated self-sufficiency of the schizoid personality often expresses an inner grandiosity reflecting severe pathological roots in the grandiose self. This brand of grandiose self-sufficiency often makes such patients relatively inaccessible to therapeutic intervention. The core difference between them may well be that the schizoid's character is taken up with a world of objects that are entirely within, whereas the narcissistic character is at least taken up with external objects, if only to the degree that they are invested with narcissistic cathexis. Schizoid character consequently must be regarded as the more severe and less treatable form of psychopathology.

Today neurotic character disorders are seen in treatment far more commonly than the symptomatic neuroses. The character disorders comprise a large portion of the population for whom analysis can be recommended. Mild schizoid characters can also be helped by analysis, but the analysis of such patients usually requires special parameters or modifications of technique, and they should never be treated by analysts who lack general psychiatric experience. This caution would probably also be advisably applied to patients who demonstrate even moderate degrees of paranoid symptomatology.

Borderline Personality Organization

The diagnosis of borderline states has only been clarified gradually in recent years. Such patients were often regarded as a variety of ambulatory schizophrenia and were frequently labeled as preschizophrenic or psychotic characters or pseudoneurotic schizophrenics. They were viewed as relatively compensated schizophrenics, who tended to regress to psychotic levels as a transient reaction to stress or to toxic influences. The present view, however, is that they represent a stable form of personality organization that is intermediate between neurotic levels of integration and the more primitive psychotic forms of personality organization.

More recent evidence seems to suggest that many borderline patients, particularly those manifesting affective lability and dysphoric tendencies, have a higher genetic affinity with primary affective disorders, even more so than with schizophrenia. The genetic disposition probably involves both affective and schizophrenic contributions in varying degrees of combination and penetrance. Borderline patients tend to have a typical constellation of symptoms and defenses and a typical pattern of defect in their object relations.

In the more primitive forms, borderline patients present a variety of neurotic symptoms and character defects. Anxiety is usually chronic and diffuse. Neurotic symptoms are multiple and include multiple phobias, obsessive thoughts and behaviors, conversion symptoms, dissociative reactions, hypochondriacal complaints, and even paranoid traits. Sexuality is frequently promiscuous and often perverse. Personality organization tends to be impulsive and infantile, and the imperative need to gratify impulses breaks through episodically, thus giving the borderline lifestyle an acting-out quality. A turning to alcohol or drugs for relief of tension and gratification is a frequent feature of this character disorder, and consequently, addictive personalities often have a borderline structure. Narcissism is often a predominant element in their character structure, and the patients frequently look clinically very much like narcissistic characters. Underlying these elements, there is often a core of paranoia based on projection of rather primitive oral rage. The underlying character dimensions may also take the form of severe depressive-masochistic pathology. The paranoid and depressive-masochistic traits are often closely related and may alternate in these patients.

The inner organization of the borderline personality reveals the weakness in the structure of the ego. These patients show a marked lack of tolerance for even low degrees of anxiety, have poor capacity for impulse control, lack suitable channels for sublimation, have a poor capacity for neutralization, and often show a generalized shift toward primary process cognitive organization. The last aspect is not usually detectable in the usual mental status examination but may be revealed on projective test material.

It is difficult for these patients to engage in a productive therapeutic relationship. Frustration tolerance is low, and narcissistic expectations and entitlements are high. The therapeutic interaction is often distorted by attempts to manipulate the therapist to gain needed gratification. The manipulation often takes the form of suicidal gesture aimed at getting the therapist to comply with the patient's wishes. Consequently, therapy with borderline patients can often be very trying and difficult. Also characteristic of the borderline personality is the intensity and chaotic quality of the transference involvement, which can alternate often quickly between excessive idealizing and dependence on the therapist, on the one hand, and devaluation of the therapist and impulsive withdrawal from therapy, on the other. This quality of the transference involvement is quite different from that found in narcissistic personalities, which often are much more remote and distant, particularly if they are caught up in needs for grandiose isolation.

A characteristic, although not exclusive, defense of the borderline patient is "splitting." This defense is also seen to a significant degree in the schizoid personalities. Splitting involves separation between good introjects, derived from satisfying object experiences, and bad introjects, derived from frustrating or rejecting object experiences. Splitting stems from a preambivalent level of development and prevents the child from integrating the objects into ambivalent (good-and-bad) objects and, correlatively, prevents the child from achieving an integration of good-and-bad internalized objects. Thus, the operations of introjection and projection maintain the internal splitting and leave the ego with a poorly developed tolerance for ambivalence—whether internal or external. There is also a correlative intolerance for anxiety. The persistence of splitting has two important consequences: First, it prevents the neutralization of aggressive drive components, and second, it provides a persistent ego defect or weakness.

From the developmental point of view, the borderline patient has not successfully reached the level of triadic oedipal conflicts that is characteristic of psychoneurotic or higher-order character disorders. The issues are more primitive and stem from preoedipal levels in

which the developmental vicissitudes of affective one-to-one relationships with the parents have been ineffectively resolved. This inability
to resolve the ambivalence toward separate parental objects prevents
their being regarded as separate and whole objects, so that the transition to the oedipal involvement is impeded. There is general agree-
ment that the level of developmental defect in borderline patients lies
somewhere in the area of separation and individuation. In 1975 Mahler
suggested that the most likely phase in which the borderline fixations
and defects occur is that of the rapprochement subphase. Among
developmental theorists, the maintenance of separate and contradictory self-configurations is thought to reflect a failure of developmental
integration and synthesis, rather than one of defensive splitting, as in
Kernberg's view.

The importance of accurate diagnosis of borderline patients cannot
be underestimated, because such patients may often present as apparently normal, or they will present with a symptomatology that amply
justifies a more benign diagnosis of neurotic personality structure.
Often the borderline features only reveal themselves after a period of
psychoanalysis or psychotherapy, when a certain amount of regression
has taken place or when the distinctive quality of the patient's object relations and their relation to splitting mechanisms becomes more
apparent.

Consequently, it is important to distinguish between levels of borderline functioning. Some borderline patients tend to maintain quite
good levels of ego functioning, to experience severe emotional difficulties in relatively restricted object-related contexts, and to regress
to levels of borderline functioning quite slowly. These patients are the
ones who may initially look neurotic or even normal and only begin to
show more borderline characteristics as a result of analytic regression.
These disorders may be regarded as higher-order forms of character
pathology within the borderline spectrum. These patients may well be
analyzable, often with the introduction of parameters or technical
modifications to the analytic situation. Other borderline patients have
more diffusely disorganized ego functioning, manifest splitting more
readily, are able to tolerate anxiety or frustration poorly, regress more
easily, and tend to act out often in destructive and self-defeating ways.
Such patients represent a lower-order organization within the borderline spectrum: they tolerate poorly the regression and object relations

conflicts inherent in analysis. Diagnosis in terms of potential analyzability in this group of patients is of primary importance.

These patients are generally not regarded as suitable for psychoanalytic treatment. Such personalities cannot generally sustain their capacity for effective therapeutic work in the face of the induced regression of the analytic situation. They often do surprisingly well, however, in a psychoanalytically oriented psychotherapeutic setting, in which they are able to establish a sufficient working alliance that involves a capacity for firm limit setting on the part of the therapist.

From a developmental perspective, the borderline patient does not have to deal primarily with the triadic oedipal issues that are characteristic of psychoneurotic patients. Rather, the issues stem from a more primitive, preoedipal level in which the developmental vicissitudes of a one-to-one relationship must be worked out. Consequently, the primary prop of the therapy of borderline patients rests on the real one-to-one relationship that is established between the therapist and the patient. The context of such a firm and trusting relationship; the difficulties of magical expectations; impairments of the distinctions between fantasy and reality; episodes of anger, suspicion, and excessive fear of rejection; and the conflicts stemming from the destructive, bad internalized objects can be gradually and productively worked through. The stability and solidity of the therapeutic alliance is important because the borderline integration is fragile and somewhat precarious, often subject to regressive pulls, and dependent on external support for its stabilization.

Perhaps the most telling and difficult area in the therapy of borderline patients is that of termination. Because of the developmental failure, the borderline patient has a limited and vulnerable capacity to internalize ego identifications. Their internalizing capacity remains more or less on an introjective level and is unable to reach the healthier and more autonomous level of identification. This basic impairment in ego capacity sets a limit on the effectiveness of therapy. Such patients may achieve considerable degrees of behavioral modification and stabilization of affect and may reach quite well-organized levels of psychic functioning and capacity for healthier and less conflicting relationships, but the capacity for regression to pretreatment levels of functioning remains a prominent element in their overall picture. In approaching the problems of termination of treatment, moreover, their markedly defective capacity for internalization impedes their capacity to separate effectively from the therapist. In analysis, treatment of such patients seems to drag on interminably. In psychotherapy, the optimal course for such patients is often a gradual attenuation of the therapeutic involvement, slowly spacing out therapeutic contact to a point where the patient is in more or less minimal, if nonetheless persistent, contact with the therapist. In a real sense, such therapies often never end.

Theory of Psychosis

Freud originally directed his attention to paranoid symptomatology as a manifestation of psychotic processes. His understanding of the mental symptoms of paranoia was greatly facilitated by the discovery of unconscious homosexuality and the mechanisms of projection. His theoretical formulations regarding this form of psychopathology were based on clinical experience to only a limited degree. He acquired considerable insight into these mechanisms, however, as a result of his careful analysis of the Schreber *Memoirs,* an autobiographical account of Schreber's paranoid psychosis and his elaborate delusional system. Schreber in fact did not recover from his paranoid decompensation and finally died in a mental asylum. Freud had never met him nor had any contact with him.

In essence, Freud's analysis of the Schreber case was an elaborate attempt to impose the basic theory of repression and return of the repressed on the paranoid material contained in Schreber's *Memoirs.* Freud postulated that, in paranoia, the need to project coincided with an unconscious impulse to homosexual love that, although of overwhelming intensity, was unconsciously denied by the patient. Thus, paranoid delusions represented sexual conflicts concerning persons of the same sex that had been projected onto some other object or force, which was then perceived as persecuting or threatening.

Other workers emphasized the close relationship of paranoid symptoms to infantile fantasies, in which feces are personalized and considered animistically as dangerous entities, which are highly powerful and destructive and threatening to the individual. In this connection the relationship between paranoia and a stage of development in which the emotions are centered on a particular part of the object's body, rather than the total person, was demonstrated by Karl Abraham. Abraham also noted that paranoid psychosis resembles certain phases of melancholia, in that the patient's fantasies indicate a desire to incorporate the object. Paranoid psychosis, however, differs from melancholia; in paranoia the hostility is directed against part of the object, rather than the whole, and the paranoid patient has fantasies that this incorporated part-object can be destroyed and eliminated by defecation.

The concurrent demonstration of the relationship of very primitive fantasies of aggression to overwhelming anxiety and the need to project has facilitated further understanding of this clinical entity. One question, however, remained unanswered: Why had the homosexuality of paranoid patients become so intense, threatening, and intolerable to the patient? This question was not examined or explained by Freud or his followers. It should be noted that more recent studies of paranoid psychosis, and even of the Schreber case itself, have tended to shift the emphasis away from homosexual dynamics and have emphasized broader and more complex issues relating to defects in ego development and dynamic conditions of primitive narcissistic traumatization, and resulting narcissistic rage, in the genesis of paranoid states.

In his classic paper "On Narcissism," Freud stated that psychosis was characterized by the patient's incapacity for normal emotional interest in other people and things. He did not feel that the psychotic process represented a total depletion of libido but, rather, that it involved a redistribution of libido that was normally devoted to object love and to self-love. The energy withdrawn from impoverished object relationships produces an abnormally excessive interest in the self, increasing the degree of cathexis of both bodily functions and the psychic attributes of the self. Concomitantly, the psychotic patient's use of language indicates a high cathectic interest in the verbal symbol, rather than in the object that the word represents. Many of the more obvious symptoms of psychosis can be considered as secondary to this primary loss of the capacity for object attachment. As Freud saw it, these are essentially rudimentary and primitive efforts to reestablish and reconstitute some degree of relationship with external objects.

Subsequent investigations have followed Freud's suggestion that the conflicts that result in psychotic adaptations occur primarily between individuals and their environment. In contrast, the conflicts character-istic of the psychoneuroses are primarily within the personality, be-tween unconscious infantile wishes and the constraining or controlling forces that adapt these wishes to the constraints and demands of re-ality. Recent work has focused more in detail on the disturbances and disorganizations in ego functioning that impair the patient's relation-ship with reality.

Psychotic states represent conditions of extreme and archaic narcis-sistic disorganization; frustration of the patient's intense narcissistic demands results in an extremely primitive, highly destructive, and po-tent narcissistic rage.

Psychotic defenses tend to be of a more primitive and narcissis-tic type, particularly denial, distortion, and projection. The primitive defenses are reflected in flight, social withdrawal, and the simple inhi-bition of impulses (blocking), which is so apparent in many psycho-tics. These defense mechanisms are much less highly organized than the higher-order mechanisms of repression or reaction formation. In contrast to the neurotic, the fear of detection by others, rather than the guilt of later childhood and maturity, is also more conspicuous in the social reactions of the psychotic.

In addition to the psychodynamic factors that are the proper realm of psychoanalytic consideration, there are most probably other con-stitutional and genetic factors that influence the basic predisposition to patterns of psychotic development. These factors are being actively studied by students of genetics, and the findings of genetic psychiatry have important and significant implications for the basic understand-ing of and ultimate capability for management of psychotic states. They do not, however, alter or minimize the significance of psycho-dynamic aspects of the psychotic process.

Analyzability

The question of analyzability is one of central importance for contemporary psychoanalysis and psychiatry. The basic question is: For what patients is psychoanalysis a suitable form of treatment? It is not uncommon for patients to develop a treatment relationship that provides relief of symptoms. By retaining the relationship with the therapist, such patients can avoid serious regression and maintain a reasonable level of adjustment and functioning. The support of ego functions, however, requires the continuing availability of the therapist.

The more difficult aspect for the treatment of such patients is the surrendering of the relationship with the therapist in termination. The patient cannot tolerate the threat of loss and separation without regression. A crucial question is the extent to which such patients are capable of internalizing and identifying with the therapist. The capacity for such internalization requires a capacity for tolerating both depressive affects and regressive forms of anxiety that might be experienced in the face of the threatened loss. Those patients who lack such capacities do not meet the criteria of analyzability.

Potentially analyzable neurotic patients have essentially been able to reach a developmental level in which a genuine triangular conflict has been experienced. They have been able to sustain significant object relations with both parents through the latency years, following on the resolution of the oedipal complex. Frequently, the postoedipal relationships between the developing neurotic and parents are less satisfactory and more ambivalent than relationships during the preoedipal periods. Moreover, the relationship with one parent during the preoedipal years generally tends to be more ambivalent than the relationship with the other parent. When the degree of ambivalence in the early mother-child relationship has been excessive, this proves to be a more severe handicap in the development of secure object relations than a highly ambivalent preoedipal relationship with the father. This distinction is applicable to both sexes. Classical psychoanalysis is the treatment of choice for potentially mature patients in whom the developmental difficulties lie on the level of the mastery of genuine internal conflicts. This implies that they have been able to establish meaningful one-to-one relationships with both parents and have been able to enter into and establish a triangular oedipal conflict. Patients who have not achieved this level of triangular involvement and conflict are generally unable to benefit from psychoanalysis.

The use of a therapeutic method that induces regression in patients who demonstrate more severe developmental failures is open to serious question. Patients who are unable to tolerate anxiety or depression are rarely able to work through a transference neurosis. The more significant difficulty for such patients is their inability to terminate successfully any form of therapy.

Patients who meet the criteria for analyzability fall into typical patterns of neurotic difficulty. The most common difficulty in analyzable women is in the area of capacities for heterosexual object relations. This is usually reflected in a hysterical form of personality organization. A more common difficulty for analyzable men is likely to be in the area of work inhibitions. Men also predominantly present with symptoms of an obsessional nature, rather than a hysterical nature. Such cases of obsessional neurosis or obsessional character usually have little difficulty in establishing the analytic situation, but few of them are able to develop the overt and analyzable transference neurosis during the first year of analysis. Considering analyzability, one must distinguish between the capacity to establish and participate in the analytic situation and the capacity to establish a genuine transference neurosis. Hysterical patients, however, present a different picture; they are either very good or very difficult patients. For them the development of a transference neurosis is relatively easy and quick, but it is more difficult for these patients to engage in and establish the analytic situation.

Freud originally noted that obsessional patients tend to develop conflicts in such important areas as love versus hate, activity versus passivity, and omnipotency versus helplessness. One can recognize today that resolution and mastery of such conflicts are crucial developmental tasks. The resolution of the conflict of love and hate, the tolerance for ambivalence, is one of the crucial developmental tasks in the achievement of healthy self-object differentiation and early identifications. This resolution determines one of the basic criteria for analyzability.

The successful analyzable obsessional patient must have sufficient tolerance for conflicting emotions to allow that patient to endure the alteration between love and hate that emerges in the transference neurosis. Further, the patient must be able to distinguish such transference feelings from the analytic relationship. In other words, patients must be sufficiently able to tolerate their ambivalence to allow themselves to maintain a real therapeutic relationship. An important distinction must be made here between the developmental failure to integrate emotions and perceptions and the regressive impairment of previously established integration during neurotic symptom formation. Obsessional intolerance for conflict and ambivalence may reflect either developmental course. Analyzable adults, however, show basic achievement in one-to-one relationships with both parents that allows the establishment of oedipal conflict to emerge without jeopardizing these important object relations.

Even so, it is quite clear that the major unresolved conflict in analyzable obsessional men derives from the triangular oedipal conflict. One can be misled, however, because obsessive reaction formations can be established in obsessional development before the onset of the genital oedipal situation. Premature consolidation of obsessional defenses and the early crystallization of personality may form an impediment to the emergence of a genuine triangular conflict. Thus, one can conclude that the presence of hysterical or obsessional systems in such patients is of much less importance in evaluating the potential for psychoanalysis than the quality of object relations and the degree to which certain major developmental steps have been accomplished.

The capacity to tolerate anxiety and depression is another of the major concerns in evaluating analyzability. Clinically, it is frequently found that obsessional characters are more vulnerable to involutional depressions toward the end of active life, but in general, depression, like hysteria, is more commonly observed in women than in men. Tolerance of depression involves a dual developmental task: (1) the passive toleration of the painful reality that cannot be immediately modified and (2) the subsequent mobilization of resources in available areas of achievement and mastery. The masculine ideal of competitive striving and mastery reinforces the second phase of this developmental task, so that it is hardly surprising that analyzable obsessional men should have a relative intolerance for passivity and depression. For women, however, passivity rather than activity is central to the image of femininity. Women may have more difficulty in dealing with the second phase of the developmental task, whereas men are more likely to have difficulty with the first phase.

In women this can lead to an exaggerated sense of passivity, helplessness, and vulnerability, characteristics found so prominently in feminine depressive character structure. This passivity may also be frequently linked with hysterical symptoms. Such women can tolerate a considerable degree of passivity and depression, but their inability to mobilize active ego resources for mastery and growth leaves them vulnerable to regression or narcissistic injury. The basic conflicts for men relate to the recognition, toleration, and integration of passivity and dependence. The transference neurosis can unmask such feelings and severely threaten the patient. Conversely, the basic conflicts for women have to do with problems related to mastery, activity, and self-assertion.

The evaluation of depression and the patient's capacity to bear and master it are crucial aspects of the evaluation for psychoanalysis. Depression is a frequent presenting symptom in patients suffering from hysterical and obsessional neurosis. Such depressed patients often turn out to be potentially analyzable neurotics. The evaluation of depression, however, is difficult and often requires a preliminary course in psychotherapy aimed at reestablishing a sufficient level of self-esteem and the mobilization of coping resources to facilitate development of a positive therapeutic alliance. The patient's therapeutic response allows the therapist to evaluate more carefully the patient's capacity to tolerate depressive affects without significant regression, as well as the patient's capacity to mobilize resources for mastery and active coping.

Analytic Process

Some of the origins of Freud's approach to treatment have been considered, particularly in the development of his basic techniques of free association and in his growing awareness and exploitation of the transference. In essence, modern psychoanalytic treatment procedures differ from those that Freud originally developed in one fundamental respect. Early in his approach to therapy, Freud felt that recognition by the physician of the patient's unconscious motivations, the communication of this knowledge to the patient, and its comprehension by the patient would of itself effect a cure. This was his basic doctrine of therapeutic insight. Further clinical experience, however, has demonstrated the fallacy of these expectations.

Specifically, Freud found that his discovery of the patient's unconscious wishes and his ability to impart these findings to the patient so that they were accepted and understood were insufficient. Such insight might permit clarification of the patient's intellectual appraisal of problems, but the emotional tensions for which the patient sought treatment were not effectively alleviated in this way. This discovery led to a significant breakthrough. Freud began to realize that the success of treatment depended on the patient's ability to understand the emotional significance of an experience on an emotional level and depended on the patient's capacity to retain and use that insight. In that event, if the experience recurred, it would elicit another reaction; it would no longer be repressed, and the patient would have undergone a psychic economic change.

Freud continually refined his technique on the basis of his expanding clinical experience and his deeper theoretical understanding, so that psychoanalysis became recognized as a specific method for reaching and modifying unconscious phenomena that give rise to conflict. More specifically, for a conflict to be considered a neurotic conflict, at least one aspect of it must be repressed. Psychoanalysis attempts to deal with repression and tries to bring the repressed material back into consciousness, so that the patient, on the basis of greater self-understanding of needs and motives, may find a more realistic solution to a conflict. Freud's formula for this process was: "Where id was, there ego shall be" (22 SE 80).

Freud thus elaborated a treatment method that attaches minimal importance to the immediate relief of symptoms, to moral support from the therapist, or to guidance. The goal of psychoanalysis is to pull the neurosis out by its roots, rather than to prune off the top. To accomplish this, it is necessary to break down the pregenital, deep crystallization of id, ego, and superego and bring the underlying material near enough to the surface of consciousness so that it can be modified and reevaluated in light of reality. This method distinguishes the classical psychoanalytic treatment from more psychodynamic forms of psychotherapy.

The repression of the forces of conflict is accomplished by design, and the patient is unaware of the psychic mechanisms the mind uses. By means of isolating the basic problem, the patient has protected against what seems, from the patient's view, to be unbearable suffering. No matter how it may impair functioning, the neurosis is somehow preferable to the emergence of unacceptable wishes and ideas. All the forces that permitted the original repression are thus mobilized once again in the analysis as a resistance to this threatened encroachment on dangerous territory. No matter how much the patient may cooperate consciously with the therapist and in the analysis, and no matter how painful the neurotic symptoms may be, the patient automatically defends against the reopening of old wounds with every subtle resource of defense and resistance available.

In discussing the analytic process, one must clarify the basic distinction between the analytic process and the analytic situation. The *analytic process* refers to the regressive emergence, working through, interpretation, and resolution of the transference neurosis. The *analytic situation*, however, refers to the setting in which the analytic process takes place, specifically the positive real relationship between patient and analyst based on the therapeutic alliance. Thus, as discussed with reference to analyzability, obsessives have difficulty with the analytic process, but have little difficulty with the analytic situation. They can easily establish and participate in the therapeutic alliance, but they experience difficulty in tolerating the regression necessary for establishing and working through the transference neurosis. Hysterics, however, have no difficulty with the analytic process, but seem to experience difficulty in the analytic situation. They find it relatively easy to regress in the analytic situation and to allow the transference neurosis to form, but they have difficulty in establishing a meaningful and secure one-to-one relationship that constitutes the therapeutic alliance.

The regression induced by the analytic situation (instinctual regression) allows for a reemergence of infantile conflicts and thus induces the formation of a transference neurosis. In the transference neurosis, the original infantile conflicts and wishes become focused on the person of the analyst and are thus reexperienced and relived. In the analytic regression, earlier infantile conflicts are revived and can be seen as a manifestation of the repetition compulsion. Regression has a dual aspect; from one point of view it is an attempt to return to an earlier state of real or fantasy gratification, but from another point of view it can be seen as an attempt to master previous traumatic experience. The regression in the analytic situation and the development of transference are preliminary conditions for the mastery of unresolved conflicts. They can also represent regressive and unconscious wishes to return to an earlier state of narcissistic gratification. The analytic process must work itself out in the face of this dual potentiality and tension.

If the analytic regression has a destructive potentiality (ego regression) that must be recognized and guarded against, it also has a progressive potentiality for reopening and reworking infantile conflicts and for achieving a reorganization and consolidation of the personality on a more mature and healthier level. As in any developmental crisis, the risk of regressive deterioration must be balanced against the promise of progressive growth and mastery. The therapeutic importance of the criteria of analyzability can be easily recognized, because patients who are unable to achieve the progressive potentiality of the analytic regression cannot be expected to realize a good therapeutic result. The determining element within the analytic situation, against which the regression must be balanced and by which the destructive or constructive potential of the regression can be measured, is the therapeutic alliance. A firm and stable alliance offers a buffer against excessive (ego) regression and also offers a basis for positive growth.

Phases of the Analytic Process

The analytic process can be usefully divided into three phases. The first phase involves the initiation and consolidation of the analytic situation. The second phase involves the emergence and analysis of the transference neurosis. The third phase involves the carrying through of a successful termination and separation from the analytic process. The three phases are important because they provide a framework for assessing the progress of the patient in analysis. Each phase of the analysis requires different capacities in the patient to successfully accomplish it, and each phase focuses on different developmental aptitudes in a patient that are required if each of the phases is to be successfully accomplished. Moreover, it is important in assessing the analyzability of a given patient to determine the relative aptitude of the patient to meet the demands of each of the respective phases.

The *first phase* relates to the patient's capacity to enter into, establish, and sustain a therapeutic alliance. This is essentially a one-to-one relationship between analyst and patient that imposes certain demands and exacts certain frustrations from the patient. The structure of the analytic situation is such that even the most mature and stable patients experience significant objective anxiety. Successful negotiation of this initial stage of the analysis involves the achievement of a special object relation that determines the nature and quality of the therapeutic alliance. The therapeutic alliance, therefore, involves both object relationship and ultimately ego identification. Both analyst and the patient are actively involved in this relationship, and it constitutes the essence of the analytic situation. The establishing of the therapeutic alliance, therefore, depends on and requires certain basic capacities in the patient. The patient must have a capacity to maintain basic trust in the absence of gratification, be able to maintain self-object differentiation in the absence of the object, retain a capacity to accept the limitations of reality, tolerate frustrations, and be able to acknowledge self-limitations and lack of omnipotence. At the same time the patient must be able to appreciate that the failure of the object to gratify wishes and demands may not be due to hostility or rejection, but may reflect realistic limitations that have to be accepted. These capacities represent a mobilization of preanalytic ego resources and are essential to establishing the therapeutic alliance.

The *second phase* of the analytic process relates to the patient's capacity to develop a genuine transference neurosis and to regress sufficiently to allow the transference neurosis to emerge and be analyzed, and to work through its respective elements. The development of the transference neurosis involves a reopening and reworking of oedipal conflicts. These basic conflicts are then relived and reexperienced in the transference and become available to the patient for interpretation and understanding. The emergence, reworking, and resolution of these conflicts involve a number of therapeutic accomplishments. Therapeutic accomplishments are paralleled by the developmental attainments in the resolution of the original conflicts. This progression involves development of a capacity to initiate and sustain intrapsychic defenses against instinctual wishes. It involves integration of both autonomous ego and ego-ideal in a capacity for positive and constructive identification with the parent of the same sex. It involves renunciation of sexualized goals in regard to the parent of the opposite sex in favor of integration of a positive object relationship with that parent. It involves neutralization or sublimation of aggressive energies mobilized in the rivalry with the parent of the same sex. The working through of the transference aims at a resolution of these basic conflicts to gain the capacity for meaningful growth inherent in the resolution of the oedipal issues.

The *third phase* involves the patient's capacity to tolerate separation and loss and to integrate these affects constructively in a pattern of positive identification with the analyst. This terminal phase of a successful analysis concerns itself more directly with the issues of autonomy and independence. To a degree, these issues have been operative through the entire course of the analysis, but they become particularly relevant in the final phase. As termination approaches, the patient's passive and dependent wishes are inevitably intensified and revivified.

The analytic task in this final phase is considerably different from that of the initial phase. In the initial phase the analyst was comparable to a parent who could respond to the regressive, passive, and dependent aspects of the infantile neurosis. In the terminal phase, however, the analyst becomes like the parent of a late adolescent who is more willing to foster and support the maturation and autonomy of the child. Passivity and dependence, so essential to the analytic regression, become increasingly ego-alien as the process continues until they come to be finally regarded as alien, infantile wishes in the terminal phase. The patient thus tends to work toward more mature acceptance of realistic limits and mobilizes personal resources to establish a more secure sense of autonomy and independence. The analyst, however, is retained as an object for continued positive identification and remains an available object, much as the good parent remains an available and supportive object for the child, even after the separation involved in growth has been accomplished.

The work of termination involves the interpretation and integration of those relatively passive components in the therapeutic alliance that can facilitate the patient's future capacity for regression in the service of the ego. The patient must surrender passive and dependent wishes. The analyst must be renounced. The patient must be able to tolerate and master the anxiety and depression involved in this renunciation. Termination is a form of mourning in which the analyst as a parent surrogate is renounced. To accomplish the work of the terminal phase, the patient must have sufficient ego resources to tolerate the pain of loss and to undertake the work of mastery necessary for a developmental gain. Also the patient must have the very important capacity to internalize the analytic situation and to identify with the positive and constructive aspects of the analyst-parent. The terminal phase of the analysis is parallel to the resolution of the oedipal situation, in which the parent must be surrendered and in which the resolution is based on the capacity for identification with the positive, ego-building aspects of the parental objects.

Treatment Techniques

The analytic technique is always adapted to the idiosyncrasies of the patient's developmental capacities, needs, and defensive constellation, as well as to the stage of the analytic process at which the patient is at any given point. The technical work of the first phase in establishing the analytic situation differs considerably from what is required in the second phase, where the regression to the transference neurosis and its resolution are involved, both of which differ considerably from the requirements imposed by the terminal phase of the analysis. Thus, the analytic techniques do not stand in isolation, but are part of a living, dynamic process that is intended to induce and achieve significant internal psychic growth.

Free Association

The cornerstone of the psychoanalytic technique is free association. The patient is taught this method and instructed to use it as well as possible throughout the treatment. The primary function of free association, besides the obvious one of providing content for the analysis, is to help to induce the necessary regression and passive dependence connected with establishing and working through the transference neurosis. Thus, free association is conjoined with the other techniques that induce such regression; namely, lying on the couch, not being able to see the analyst, and conducting the analysis in an atmosphere of quiet and restful tranquillity.

The use of free association in the analytic process is a relative matter. Although it remains the basic technique and the fundamental rule by which the patient's participation in the analysis is guided, there are multiple and frequent occasions in which the process of free association is interrupted, or modified, according to the defensive needs or the developmental progression taking place within the analysis. The analyst is never in the position of simply passively listening to the endless free associations of the patient. The older model of the analyst as the passive mirror of the patient's associations is no longer functional and can now be recognized as an unrealistic and unproductive distortion of the analytic process.

One also cannot simply regard the process of free association as something that takes place in isolation in the patient. In fact the process is more complex, more difficult to conceptualize, and increasingly must be seen in the context of and in reference to the more fundamental relationship between analyst and patient. The patient's free associating is a function of the more basic relationship. Moreover, it is increasingly clear from a contemporary perspective that much more is required of a patient than the act of simply free associating. It is not enough for the patient to lie back and allow self-surrender to a position of passive dependency within the analytic relationship, without at the same time being required to mobilize basic ego resources in the service of mastery, gaining insight, mobilizing executive and synthetic capacities, and ultimately being able to assume a less passive and more active function within the analytic relationship. Obviously, there is a gradation in the mobilization of these capacities in the patient, which varies from phase to phase of the analytic process.

Resistance

The most conscientious efforts on the part of the patient to say everything that comes to mind are never completely successful. No matter how willing and cooperative the patient is in attempting to free associate, the signs of resistance are apparent throughout the course of every analysis. The patient pauses abruptly, corrects himself or herself, makes a slip of the tongue, stammers, remains silent, fidgets with some part of clothing, or asks irrelevant questions, intellectualizes, arrives late for appointments, finds excuses for not keeping them, offers critical evaluations of the rationale underlying the treatment method, simply cannot think of anything to say, or even censors thoughts that do occur and decides that they are banal or uninteresting or irrelevant and not worth mentioning.

The development of resistance in the analysis is quite as automatic and independent of the patient's will as the development of the transference itself. The sources of the resistance are just as unconscious as the sources of the transference. The emotional forces, however, that give rise to resistance are opposed to those that tend to produce the transference neurosis. Thus, the role of resistance in the analysis is particularly focused in the second phase, in which the regressive emergence of the transference is a central concern. The analysis becomes a recurring conflict between the tendencies toward transference and those toward resistance, manifested by the involuntary inhibition of the patient's efforts to associate freely. This inhibition may last for moments or days or may persist through the whole course of the analysis.

Resistance may take place in the other phases of analysis, but its quality and its significance are different in those phases, depending on the analytic task at hand. In any case, the resistance offered in the analysis enables the analyst to evaluate and become familiar with the defensive organization of the patient's ego and its functions. In this way the pattern of resistance not only offers valuable information to the analyst but also offers a channel by which the patient can be approached therapeutically. Part of the work of the second phase is the working through of resistance and defenses in the interest of facilitating the regression to a transference neurosis. In helping the patient to gradually discover and work through defenses, it is inevitable that the patient and analyst together come close to understanding what it is in fact that the patient must defend against.

The significance of this basic conflict is clear. It is a repetition of the very same sexuality-guilt conflict that originally produced the neurosis itself. Transference may itself be a form of resistance, in that the wish for immediate gratification in the analysis can circumvent and postpone the essential goals of treatment. The wish for immediate gratification runs counter to the demands for tolerance of anxiety, delay of gratification, mastery, and growth, which are basic to the analytic process. Consequently, the analysis of resistance, particularly transference resistance, constitutes a primary function of the analyst. It also accounts in many cases for the extended time period required for successful psychoanalytic treatment.

No matter how skillful the analyst, resistance is never absent. The character of the resistance tends to change from phase to phase of the analysis. In the initial phase, the patient's resistance may be directed toward establishing the analytic situation and entering into a real one-to-one and meaningful relationship with the analyst. In the second phase, resistance is usually more concerned with keeping the underlying conflicts unconscious and working against the induced regression of the analytic process. In this phase, resistance tends to inhibit and postpone the emergence and development of a transference. In the terminal phase, however, resistance often takes an opposite tack in that it works in the interest of clinging to the passive and dependent and relatively regressed relationship with the analyst, thus resisting the demands of the terminal phase to activate resources for mastery and growth and the necessity of taking a more autonomous and independent stand in relationship to the analyst and the analytic process.

Interpretation

Interpretation is the chief tool available to the analyst in the efforts to reduce unconscious resistance. As mentioned earlier, in the early stages of the development of psychoanalytic therapeutic techniques, the sole purpose of interpretation was to inform the patient of his or her unconscious wishes. Later, it was designed to help the patient understand the resistance to spontaneous and helpful self-awareness. In current psychoanalytic practice, the analyst's function as interpreter is not limited to simply paraphrasing the patient's verbal reports but, rather, to indicating at appropriate moments what is not reported. Consequently, as a general rule, analytic interpretation does not produce immediate symptomatic relief. On the contrary, there may be a heightening of anxiety and an emergence of further resistance.

If a correct interpretation is given at the proper time (mutative interpretation), the patient may react either immediately or after a period of emotional struggle during which new associations are offered. These new associations often confirm the validity of previous interpretations and add significant additional data, thus disclosing motivations and experiences of the patient of which the analyst could not previously have been aware. Generally speaking, it is not so much the analyst's insight into the patient's psychodynamics that produces progress in the analysis as it is the ability to help the patient to gain this insight independently, by reducing unconscious resistance to such self-awareness through appropriate, carefully timed interpretation. The most effective interpretation is timed so that it is given by the analyst in such a way as to meet the emerging, if hesitant and half-formed, awareness of the patient. Thus, the analyst must gauge the capacity of the patient at any given moment to hear, assimilate, and integrate the content of a given interpretation.

Another important aspect of interpretations is that they cannot be seen in isolation from the total context of the analytic situation and the analytic process. An interpretation, both as given by the analyst and as received by the patient—and that includes the elements of transference neurosis and therapeutic alliance—takes place within the context of the therapeutic relationship. Thus, the giving and receiving of interpretations are cloaked with a series of meanings that unavoidably influence both the capacity of the patient to accept and integrate interpretations and the analyst's sense of offering and providing such interpretations. Experience has shown that, at best, the therapeutic benefits produced by virtue of the analyst's exhortations or unilaterally provided insights are only temporary. Those interpretations are most effective and of lasting therapeutic value that are arrived at by the delicate dialectic arising from the mutually facilitated and growing awareness of both patient and analyst.

Role of the Analyst

The role of the analyst in the analytic process can be understood specifically in relation to the phases of analysis and the related developmental problems at issue in each of the respective phases. In the initial phase of the analysis, the analyst's task is to facilitate the establishing of the analytic situation and the therapeutic alliance. With healthier patients this is generally not a difficult feature of the analysis. These patients are capable of entering into a trusting and productive working relationship with the analyst without any great difficulty.

In the beginning the quality of the patient's interaction with the analyst is more a function of the dimensions of the patient's viable personality and the interaction with characteristics of the analyst's personality than it is a function of regressive transference elements. Unquestionably, in most analytic patients, transference elements are at work almost from the beginning, but other more realistic aspects of the patient's personality and the interaction with the analyst must be taken into account and given consideration. In more hysterical patients, particularly, as well as in patients who develop a transference readiness before the beginning of the analysis itself, there may be a tendency to move more quickly into transference issues, in which case the analyst must help the patient build the foundations for a firm therapeutic alliance. The more severe the level of psychopathology in general, the more significant and important is the work of the first phase. Where the therapeutic alliance is firmly and securely established, the more regressive aspects of the treatment situation can be faced with greater confidence and less risk of harmful regression. Where the therapeutic relationship is not so established, the risk in regression is greater.

In the transition to the middle phase of analysis, which concerns itself much more directly with transference neurosis, the analyst's role becomes closer to the traditional model in that the analyst uses the approaches and techniques calculated to induce greater regression in the patient. If the analyst's focus in the initial phases of analysis has been primarily on the real aspects of the patient's interaction and feelings, while maintaining a certain objectivity and distance in dealing with repressed instinctual derivatives, in the second phase the analyst must become more like the parent who can recognize the child's incestuous fantasies without gratifying them.

The transference regression involves a recapitulation of crucial aspects of the mother-child relationship. In the beginning of the analytic process, the analyst is like a mother adapting to the innate dispositions of her child. Responses to the patient are intuitively adaptive and are calculated to mobilize the patient's resources in the service of establishing a real relationship. In the second phase of the analysis the relative passivity of the analyst implies the avoidance of permissive, as well as authoritative, expressions and allows self-limitation to interpretations, offered at the proper time, of the patient's mental dynamics as these emerge in free associations. It also allows the analyst to clarify the way in which the patient's ego defense mechanisms operate to inhibit or preclude free association, thus preventing insight into unconscious wishes and impulses. In this respect, the passive role of the analyst reduces the realistic features of the patient-physician relationship that has been the primary focus of the initial phase of the analysis.

The analyst's task in the second phase is to maintain the stabilizing therapeutic alliance but to facilitate the regression to a transference neurosis. The work of interpretation in this context has to do with the understanding of and working through of infantile conflicts derived from the infantile neurosis. One of the important aspects of this working through has to do with the differentiation between the therapeutic alliance and the elements of the transference neurosis. The therapeutic alliance enables the patient to differentiate between the objective reality of the alliance and the distortions and projections of the transference. The patient must be able to appreciate the difference between the reality of the personality characteristics of the analyst as a real object and the transference distortions that derive from the infantile neurosis. The therapeutic process therefore involves a dual approach. The analyst must respond to the patient both in terms of the transference material and in terms of the therapeutic alliance. While also continuing to respond intuitively to the patient's affect, particularly the basic need to feel accepted and understood as a real person, the analyst must recognize and interpret any wishes or fantasies derived from the transference neurosis.

Dynamics of the Therapeutic Process

In the course of analysis, the patient undergoes two processes, remembering and reliving, that constitute the dynamics of the treatment process. Remembering refers to the gradual extension of consciousness back to early childhood, at which time the core of the neurosis was formed, for this stage of development marked the onset of the interference and distortion of the patient's instinctual life. Consequently, making the unconscious conscious is accomplished in part by the recovery of these events. More often, however, the recovery is made in other ways through the use of fantasy, inference, and analogy. In successfully analyzed patients this means more than mere verbal autobiographical reconstruction. Inevitably, inner convictions and values that were formed in early life will be reevaluated and altered so they can contribute to, rather than hinder, the patient's optimal functioning. Reliving refers to the actual reexperiencing of these events in the context of the patient's relationship with the analyst.

Transference
Through free association, hidden patterns of the patient's mental organization that fixated at immature levels are brought to life, com-

paratively free from disguise. These free associations refer to events or fantasies that are part of the patient's private experience. When they are shared in the analytic setting, the analyst is gradually invested with some of the emotions that accompany them. The patient displaces the feelings originally directed toward the earlier objects onto the analyst, who then becomes alternately a friend or enemy, one who is nice or frustrates needs and punishes, one who is loved or hated, as the original objects were loved or hated. Moreover, this tendency persists, so that to an increasing extent the patient's feelings toward the analyst replicate feelings toward the specific people being talked about or, more accurately, those about whom the patient's unconscious is talking. This special type of object displacement that is an inevitable concomitant of psychoanalytic treatment is referred to as "transference."

As unresolved childhood attitudes emerge and begin to function as fantasied projections toward the analyst, he or she becomes for the patient a phantom composite figure who represents various important persons in the patient's early environment. Those earlier relationships that remain unresolved are reactivated with some of their original vigor. Gradually, patients see themselves as they really are, with all unfulfilled and contradictory needs spread before them. The conscious, scientific use of transference as a dynamic therapeutic force through the analysis of its unconscious sources is unique to classical psychoanalysis. The combination of these two processes—remembering and reliving—enables patients to gain deeper insights into the defects of their psychological functioning, in spite of themselves.

Transference Neurosis

The transference neurosis usually develops in the second phase of analysis. The patient who at first was eager for improved mental health no longer consistently displays such motivation during the treatment hours. Rather, the patient is engaged in a continuing battle with the analyst, and it becomes apparent that the most compelling reason for continuing analysis is the desire to attain some kind of emotional satisfaction from the analyst. At this point of the treatment, the transference emotions are more important to the patient than the permanent health sought initially. It is at this point that the major, unresolved, unconscious problems of childhood begin to dominate the patient's behavior. They are now reproduced in the transference, with all their pent-up emotion. The patient is striving unconsciously to recapture what was actually taken away in childhood.

The transference neurosis is governed by three outstanding characteristics of instinctual life in early childhood: the pleasure principle (before effective reality testing), ambivalence, and repetition compulsion. The emergence of the transference neurosis in the analytic setting is usually a slow and gradual process, although in certain patients with a propensity for transference regression, particularly the more hysterical patients, the elements of the transference and the transference neurosis may manifest themselves relatively early in the analytic process. The full comprehension and management of the transference neurosis are tests of skill that sharply differentiate those analysts who have received adequate training in classical psychoanalytic theory and technique from those who have not.

One situation after another in the life of the patient is analyzed until the original infantile conflict is fully revealed. Only then does the transference neurosis begin to subside. At that point the juncture between the second phase and third phase of analysis is marked. Termination of the analysis begins from that point. However, it is a gradual process that is not even complete with the last visit to the analyst. If, however, exposure of the unconscious source of the patient's major problem was fairly thorough, at times of emotional crisis thereafter the patient may resolve, through association and without assistance, those areas of conflict that were not entirely worked through with the analyst. Part of the patient's capacity to do this depends on the capacity for internalization and effective identification with the strength and objectivity of the analyst. After a variable period, the temporarily accentuated awareness of the unconscious diminishes. Useful repressions are then partially reestablished. The patient experiences less need for introspection and self-analysis and is gradually more able to deal with life on a more mature and satisfactory basis than was possible previously.

Therapeutic Alliance

The therapeutic alliance is based on the one-to-one collaborative relationship that the patient establishes in the interaction with the analyst. This interaction is contributed to by the real personality characteristics of both the patient and the analyst. The distortions or misperceptions that the patient brings to this relationship may not all be due to transference but may be determined by the relatively stable aspects of the patient's personality structure that relate more directly to the capacity to achieve and maintain a stable object relationship.

For this reason the analyst's attempts to clarify the patient's anxiety, suspicions, fears, and unrealistic hopes and expectations, or feelings about the analyst, particularly in the beginning of the analytic process, should not be regarded as transference interpretations. The purpose of such analytic interventions is to support and reinforce the patient's capacity to enter and establish a meaningful therapeutic alliance. The importance of the therapeutic alliance cannot be underestimated because it provides the stable and positive relationship between analyst and patient that enables them both to productively engage in the work of analysis. This therapeutic alliance allows a split to take place in the patient's ego; that is, the observing part of the patient's ego can ally itself with the analyst in a working relationship, which allows it to gradually identify positively with the analyst in analyzing and modifying the pathological defenses put up by the defensive ego against internal danger situations. The maintenance of this therapeutic split, as well as the real relationship to the analyst involved in the therapeutic alliance, requires the maintenance of self-object differentiation, tolerance and mastery of ambivalence, and the capacity to distinguish fantasy from reality in the relationship.

The analyst's own personality has an important influence in establishing the therapeutic alliance. The analyst enters the analytic process as a real person and not merely as a transference object. Recognizing this aspect of the analytic situation, it should be clearly differentiated from excessive activity or inappropriate participation in the analytic relationship by the analyst. It should be recognized nonetheless that the analyst's real characteristics can interfere with the achieving of a basic working relationship and that this impediment to the therapeutic alliance can interfere with the satisfactory working through in the analytic process. The maintenance of the therapeutic alliance requires that the patient be able to differentiate between the more mature and the more infantile aspects of the experience in the relationship to the analyst. The therapeutic alliance serves a double function. On one hand, it acts as a significant barrier to regression of the ego in the analytic process; on the other hand, it serves as a fundamental aspect of the analytic situation, against which the wishes, feelings, and fantasies evoked by the transference neurosis can be evaluated and measured. In many pathological conditions—some character neuroses, border-line personalities, and the more severe neurotic disorders—it may be impossible to maintain a clinical distinction between therapeutic alliance as a real object relationship and the transference neurosis.

The therapeutic alliance derives from the mobilization of specific ego resources relating to the capacity for object relations and reality testing. The analyst must direct attention toward eliciting the patient's capacity to establish such a relationship that will be able to withstand the inevitable distortions and regressive aspects of the transference neurosis. The ego capacities involved are closely related to the resolution of pregenital conflicts, and the relationship that forms the basis of the therapeutic alliance must itself be included in the transference analysis.

It is inevitable that the fundamental features of the therapeutic alliance be carefully evaluated and understood and ultimately integrated with the analysis of the transference neurosis. This point is particularly and graphically displayed in the analysis of hysterical patients. The initial transference neurosis of such patients tends to present primarily oedipal material, but analysts have learned to appreciate the importance of underlying oral factors in the genesis of hysterical disorders. In the terminal stages of analysis of these patients, it becomes increasingly clear that resolution of oedipal conflicts depends on the successful analysis of earlier conflicts stemming from the pregenital level of development. Specifically involved are conflicts, usually on an oral level, that are related to achieving early object relations and the acceptance of reality and its limitations. These elements, however, are specifically those that form the developmental basis of the therapeutic alliance.

Modifications in Techniques

There are no shortcuts in psychoanalytic treatment. Psychoanalytic treatment typically extends over a period of years and requires interminable patience on the part of both the physician and the patient. The classical analytic method, which best serves the aims of therapy,

also constitutes the best experimental situation yet devised for studying the more complex features of human nature.

Rigid adherence, however, at all times to the fundamental mecha-
nistic principles of psychoanalytic technique is an impossibility. For
example, the immediate environmental situation may be so serious
for the patient that the analyst must pay commonsense attention to
its practical implications. Those patients whose early childhood was
extraordinarily deficient in love and affection, so that they suffer from
a basic developmental defect in their capacity for one-to-one relationship and, consequently, in their capacity to sustain a therapeutic alliance, must be given more support and encouragement than is advo-
cated by strict psychoanalytic technique.

The analyst's role in the early stages of analysis in helping to establish the therapeutic alliance is of particular importance. As noted, with
the primitive patients the establishing of a therapeutic alliance can be
the more significant aspect of the treatment process and can even persist as a problem through most of the analysis. The establishing of the
therapeutic alliance for most patients is a significant aspect of the analytic process.

The nature and the degree of the analyst's active intervention in
the opening hours of analysis are still matters of considerable discussion and controversy. The transference neurosis usually develops only
gradually, so that attempts at premature interpretation in the early
hours may not be productive and may even be counterproductive. This
has tended to foster the use of prolonged silences, lack of responsiveness, rigidity, and relative lack of participation in the analysis on the
part of the analyst, as if any reference to the analytic situation or to the
person of the analyst or to the patient's feelings about the analyst was
to be taken as a transference interpretation and thus to be avoided.
Often, however, serious problems in the subsequent stages of analysis
of the transference can be due to a failure to establish a meaningful alliance in the initial stages of treatment. Thus, suitable interventions of
the analyst in the early stages of treatment can be a help to the patient
in establishing such a meaningful therapeutic alliance.

Patients who are more borderline or very narcissistic must establish
a strong personal tie and strong feelings of attachment and relationship with the analyst before they can develop sufficient interest and

motivation for treatment. Moreover, such a strong object tie and alliance with the analyst for these more primitive patients is an absolute necessity if the destructive effects of excessive regression are to
be avoided. These are difficult problems, however, because experience
also suggests that every deviation from strict analytic technique that
such special conditions compel tends to prolong the length of treatment and to considerably increase its vicissitudes and problems.

Such modifications in analytic technique usually go under the heading of "parameters," and they remain a considerable source of discussion and controversy among analytic therapists. A significant trend
today is the increasing tendency of analysts to treat more difficult and
complex cases; thus, the necessity for introducing modifications in
various aspects of the treatment process correspondingly increases.
The resolution of such difficulties in assessing and exploring modifications of techniques must ultimately rest on the basis of clinical experience.

Results of Treatment

The therapeutic effectiveness of psychoanalysis presents problems in its evaluation. Impartial and objective critics are handicapped
in attempts to appraise therapeutic results by the fact that so many patients state that they have been analyzed when no such procedure was,
in fact, undertaken or when it was undertaken by someone who used
the title of analyst and who, in fact, had little understanding of analytic science and technique. Other patients have been in analysis only
for a very short time and then discontinued treatment on their own
initiative or were advised they were not suitable candidates for analytic treatment. Except for psychoanalysts themselves, professionals as
well as laypeople demonstrate varying degrees of confusion as to what
psychoanalysis is and what it is not.

No analyst can ever eliminate all the personality defects and neurotic factors in a given patient, no matter how thorough or successful
the treatment. Mitigation of the rigors of a punitive superego, however, is an essential criterion of the effectiveness of treatment. Psychoanalysts do not usually regard alleviation of symptoms as the most
significant aspect in evaluating therapeutic change. The absence of
a recurrence of the illness or a further need for psychotherapy is per-

haps a more important index of the value of psychoanalysis. The chief basis of evaluation, however, remains the patient's general adjustment to life; that is, the capacity for attaining reasonable happiness, for contributing to the happiness of others, the ability to deal adequately with the normal vicissitudes and stresses of life, and the capacity to enter into and sustain mutually gratifying and rewarding relationships with other people in the patient's life.

More specific criteria of the effectiveness of treatment include the reduction of the patient's unconscious, neurotic need for suffering, reduction of neurotic inhibitions, decrease of infantile dependency needs, and an increased capacity for responsibility, for successful relationships in marriage, work, and social relations. Other important criteria are the capacity for pleasurable and rewarding sublimation and for creative and adaptive application of the patient's own potentialities. The most important criterion of the success of treatment, however, is the release of the patient's normal potentiality, which had been blocked by neurotic conflicts, for further internal growth, development, and maturation to mature personality functioning.

Appendix

Table A.   Stages of Psychosexual Development

Oral Stage

Definition	The earliest stage of development in which the infant's needs, perceptions, and modes of expression are primarily centered in the mouth, lips, tongue, and other organs related to the oral zone.
Description	The oral zone maintains its dominant role in the organization of the psyche through approximately the first 18 months of life. Oral sensations include thirst, hunger, pleasurable tactile stimulations evoked by the nipple or its substitute, sensations related to swallowing and satiation. Oral drives consist of two separate components: libidinal and aggressive. States of oral tension lead to a seeking for oral gratification, typified by quiescence at the end of nursing. The oral triad consists of the wish to eat, to sleep, and to reach that relaxation that occurs at the end of sucking just before the onset of sleep. Libidinal needs (oral erotism) are thought to predominate in the early parts of the oral phase, whereas they are mixed with more aggressive components later (oral sadism). Oral aggression may express itself in biting, chewing, spitting, or crying. Oral aggression is connected with primitive wishes and fantasies of biting, devouring, and destroying.
Objectives	To establish a trusting dependence on nursing and sustaining objects, to establish comfortable expression and gratification of oral libidinal needs without excessive conflict or ambivalence from oral sadistic wishes.
Pathological traits	Excessive oral gratifications or deprivation can result in libidinal fixations that contribute to pathological traits. Such traits can include excessive optimism, narcissism, pessimism (often seen in depressive states), or demandingness. Oral characters are often excessively dependent and require others to give to them and to look after them. Such individuals want to be fed, but may be exceptionally giving to elicit a return of being given to. Oral characters are often extremely dependent on objects for the maintenance of their self-esteem. Envy and jealousy are often associated with oral traits.
Character traits	Successful resolution of the oral phase provides a basis in character structure for capacities to give to and receive from others without excessive dependence or envy. A capacity to rely on others with a sense of trust as well as with a sense of self-reliance and self-trust.

Table A.   Stages of Psychosexual Development (*cont.*)

Anal Stage

Definition	The stage of psychosexual development that is prompted by maturation of neuromuscular control over sphincters, particularly the anal sphincters, thus permitting more voluntary control over retention or expulsion of feces.
Description	This period, which extends roughly from 1 to 3 years of age, is marked by a recognizable intensification of aggressive drives mixed with libidinal components, in sadistic impulses. Acquisition of voluntary sphincter control is associated with an increasing shift from passivity to activity. The conflicts over anal control and the struggle with the parent over retaining or expelling feces in toilet training give rise to increased ambivalence, together with a struggle over separation, individuation, and independence. Anal erotism refers to the sexual pleasure in anal functioning, both in retaining the precious feces and in presenting them as a precious gift to the parent. Anal sadism refers to the expression of aggressive wishes connected with discharging feces as powerful and destructive weapons. These wishes are often displayed in such children's fantasies as bombing or explosions.
Objectives	The anal period is essentially a period of striving for independence and separation from the dependence on and control of the parent. The objectives of sphincter control without overcontrol (fecal retention) or loss of control (messing) are matched by the child's attempts to achieve autonomy and independence without excessive shame or self-doubt from loss of control.
Pathological traits	Maladaptive character traits, often apparently inconsistent, are derived from anal erotism and the defenses against it. Orderliness, obstinacy, stubbornness, willfulness, frugality, and parsimony are features of the anal character derived from a fixation on anal functions. When defenses against anal traits are less effective, the anal character reveals traits of heightened ambivalence, lack of tidiness, messiness, defiance, rage, and sadomasochistic tendencies. Anal characteristics and defenses are most typically seen in obsessive-compulsive neuroses.
Character traits	Successful resolution of the anal phase provides the basis for the development of personal autonomy, a capacity for independence and personal initiative without guilt, a capacity for self-determining behavior without a sense of shame or self-doubt, a lack of ambivalence and a capacity for willing cooperation without either excessive willfulness or sense of self-diminution or defeat.

Table A.   Stages of Psychosexual Development (*cont.*)

Urethral Stage

Definition	This stage was not explicitly treated by Freud but is envisioned as a transitional stage between the anal and phallic stages of development. It shares some of the characteristics of the preceding anal phase and some from the subsequent phallic phase.
Description	The characteristics of the urethral phase are often subsumed under those of the phallic phase. Urethral erotism, however, is used to refer to the pleasure in urination as well as the pleasure in urethral retention analogous to anal retention. Similar issues of performance and control are related to urethral functioning. Urethral functioning may also be invested with a sadistic quality, often reflecting the persistence of anal sadistic urges. Loss of urethral control, as in enuresis, may frequently have regressive significance that reactivates anal conflicts.
Objectives	Issues of control and urethral performance and loss of control. It is not clear whether or to what extent the objectives of urethral functioning differ from those of the anal period.
Pathological traits	The predominant urethral trait is that of competitiveness and ambition, probably related to the compensation for shame due to loss of urethral control. In control this may be the start for development of penis envy, related to the feminine sense of shame and inadequacy in being unable to match the male urethral performance. This is also related to issues of control and shaming.
Character traits	Besides the healthy effects analogous to those from the anal period, urethral competence provides a sense of pride and self-competence derived from performance. Urethral performance is an area in which the small boy can imitate and match his father's more adult performance. The resolution of urethral conflicts sets the stage for budding gender identity and subsequent identifications.

Table A. Stages of Psychosexual Development (*cont.*)

Phallic Stage

Definition	The phallic stage of sexual development begins sometime during the third year of life and continues until approximately the end of the fifth year.
Description	The phallic phase is characterized by a primary focus of sexual interests, stimulation, and excitement in the genital area. The penis becomes the organ of principal interest to children of both sexes, with the lack of penis in the female being considered as evidence of castration. The phallic phase is associated with an increase in genital masturbation accompanied by predominantly unconscious fantasies of sexual involvement with the opposite-sex parent. The threat of castration and its related castration anxiety arise in connection with guilt over masturbation and oedipal wishes. During this phase the oedipal involvement and conflict are established and consolidated.
Objectives	The objective of this phase is to focus erotic interest in the genital area and genital functions. This focusing lays the foundation for gender identity and serves to integrate the residues of previous stages of psychosexual development into a predominantly genital-sexual orientation. The establishing of the oedipal situation is essential for the furtherance of subsequent identifications that will serve as the basis for important and perduring dimensions of character organization.
Pathological traits	The derivation of pathological traits from the phallic-oedipal involvement are sufficiently complex and subject to such a variety of modifications that it encompasses nearly the whole of neurotic development. The issues, however, focus on castration in males and on penis envy in females. The other important focus of developmental distortions in this period derives from the patterns of identification which are developed out of the resolution of the oedipal complex. The influence of castration anxiety and penis envy, the defenses against both of these, and the patterns of identification that emerge from the phallic phase are the primary determinants of the development of human character. They also subsume and integrate the residues of previous psychosexual stages, so that fixations or conflicts that derive from any of the preceding stages can contaminate and modify the oedipal resolution.

Table A.   Stages of Psychosexual Development (*cont.*)

Phallic Stage (cont.)

Character traits	The phallic stage provides the foundations for an emerging sense of sexual identity, of a sense of curiosity without embarrassment, of initiative without guilt, as well as a sense of mastery not only over objects and persons in the environment but also over internal processes and impulses. The resolution of the oedipal conflict at the end of the phallic period gives rise to powerful internal resources for regulation of drive impulses and their direction to constructive ends. This internal source of regulation is the superego, and it is based on identifications derived primarily from parental figures.

Latency Stage

Definition	The stage of relative quiescence or inactivity of the sexual drive during the period from the resolution of the Oedipus complex until pubescence (from about 5–6 years until about 11–13 years).
Description	The institution of the superego at the close of the oedipal period and the further maturation of ego functions allow for a considerably greater degree of control of instinctual impulses. Sexual interests during this period are generally thought to be quiescent. This is a period of primarily homosexual affiliations for both boys and girls, as well as a sublimation of libidinal and aggressive energies into energetic learning and play activities, exploring the environment, and becoming more proficient in dealing with the world of things and persons around them. It is a period for development of important skills. The relative strength of regulatory elements often gives rise to patterns of behavior that are somewhat obsessive and hypercontrolling.

Table A.   Stages of Psychosexual Development (*cont.*)

Latency Stage (cont.)

Objectives	The primary objective in this period is the further integration of oedipal identifications and a consolidation of sex-role identity and sex roles. The relative quiescence and control of instinctual impulses allow for development of ego apparatuses and mastery skills. Further identificatory components may be added to the oedipal ones on the basis of broadening contacts with other significant figures outside the family, e.g., teachers, coaches, and other adult figures.
Pathological traits	The danger in the latency period can arise either from a lack of development of inner controls or an excess of them. The lack of control can lead to a failure of the child to sufficiently sublimate energies in the interests of learning and development of skills; an excess of inner control, however, can lead to premature closure of personality development and the precocious elaboration of obsessive character traits.
Character traits	The latency period has frequently been regarded as a period of relatively unimportant inactivity in the developmental schema. More recently, greater respect has been gained for the developmental processes that take place in this period. Important consolidations and additions are made to the basic postoedipal identifications. It is a period of integrating and consolidating previous attainments in psychosexual development and of establishing decisive patterns of adaptive functioning. The child can develop a sense of industry and a capacity for mastery of objects and concepts that allows autonomous function and with a sense of initiative without running the risk of failure or defeat or a sense of inferiority. These are all important attainments that need to be further integrated, ultimately as the essential basis for a mature adult life of satisfaction in work and love.

Table A.   Stages of Psychosexual Development (*cont.*)

Genital Stage

Definition   The genital or adolescent phase of psychosexual development
              extends from the onset of puberty from ages 11–13 until the in-
              dividual reaches young adulthood. In current thinking, there
              is a tendency to subdivide this stage into preadolescent, early
              adolescent, middle adolescent, late adolescent, and even
              postadolescent periods.

Description   The physiological maturation of systems of genital (sexual)
              functioning and attendant hormonal systems leads to an in-
              tensification of drives, particularly libidinal drives. This pro-
              duces a regression in personality organization, which reopens
              conflicts of previous stages of psychosexual development and
              provides the opportunity for a reresolution of these conflicts
              in the context of achieving a mature sexual and adult identity.

Objectives   The primary objectives of this period are the ultimate separa-
              tion from dependence on and attachment to the parents and
              the establishment of mature, nonincestuous, heterosexual ob-
              ject relations. Related to this are the achievement of a mature
              sense of personal identity and acceptance and integration of a
              set of adult roles and functions that permit new adaptive inte-
              grations with social expectations and cultural values.

Pathological The pathological deviations due to a failure to achieve success-
traits   ful resolution of this stage of development are multiple and
              complex. Defects can arise from the whole spectrum of psy-
              chosexual residues, since the developmental task of the ado-
              lescent period is in a sense a partial reopening and reworking
              and reintegrating of all of these aspects of development. Pre-
              vious unsuccessful resolutions and fixations in various phases
              or aspects of psychosexual development will produce patho-
              logical defects in the emerging adult personality. A more
              specific defect from a failure to resolve adolescent issues has
              been described by Erikson as "identity diffusion."

Character   The successful resolution and reintegration of previous psy-
traits   chosexual stages in the adolescent, fully genital phase, sets the
              stage normally for a fully mature personality with a capacity
              for full and satisfying genital potency and a self-integrated and
              consistent sense of identity. Such an individual has reached a
              satisfying capacity for self-realization and meaningful partici-
              pation in areas of work, love, and in the creative and produc-
              tive application to satisfying and meaningful goals and values.
              Only in the last few years has the presumed relationship be-
              tween psychosexual genitality and maturity of personality
              functioning been put in question.

Table B.   Classification of Defense Mechanisms*

Narcissistic Defenses

Projection	Perceiving and reacting to unacceptable inner impulses and their derivatives as though they were outside the self. On a psychotic level, this takes the form of frank delusions about external reality, usually persecutory, includes both perception of one's own feelings in another, with subsequent acting on the perception (psychotic paranoid delusions). The impulses may derive from the id or superego (hallucinated recriminations) but may undergo transformation in the process. Thus, according to Freud's analysis of paranoid projections, homosexual libidinal impulses are transformed into hatred and then projected onto the object of the unacceptable homosexual impulse.
Denial	Psychotic denial of external reality, unlike repression, affects the perception of external reality more than the perception of internal reality. Seeing, but refusing to acknowledge what one sees, or hearing, and negating what is actually heard, are examples of denial and exemplify the close relationship of denial to sensory experience. Not all denial, however, is necessarily psychotic. Like projection, denial may function in the service of more neurotic or even adaptive objectives. Denial avoids becoming aware of some painful aspect of reality. At the psychotic level, the denied reality may be replaced by a fantasy or delusion.
Distortion	Grossly reshaping external reality to suit inner needs, including unrealistic megalomaniac beliefs, hallucinations, wish-fulfilling delusions, and employing sustained feelings of delusional superiority or entitlement.

Immature Defenses

Acting Out	The direct expression of an unconscious wish or impulse in action to avoid being conscious of the accompanying affect. The unconscious fantasy, involving objects, is lived out impulsively in behavior, thus gratifying the impulse more than the prohibition against it. On a chronic level, acting out involves giving in to impulses to avoid the tension that would result from postponement of expression.

* Compiled and adapted from Semrad (1967), Bibring et al. (1961), and Vaillant (1971).

Table B.   Classification of Defense Mechanisms (*cont.*)

Immature Defenses (cont.)

Blocking   An inhibition, usually temporary in nature, of affects es-
                     pecially, but possibly also thinking and impulses. It is close
                     to repression in its effects, but has a component of ten-
                     sion arising from the inhibition of the impulse, affect, or
                     thought.

Hypochondriasis   The transformation of reproach toward others arising from
                     bereavement, loneliness, or unacceptable aggressive im-
                     pulses, into self-reproach and complaints of pain, somatic
                     illness. and neurasthenia. Existent illness may also be over-
                     emphasized or exaggerated for its evasive and regressive
                     possibilities. Thus, responsibility may be avoided, guilt may
                     be circumvented, instinctual impulses may be warded off.

Introjection   In addition to the developmental functions of the process
                     of introjection, it also serves specific defensive functions.
                     The introjection of a loved object involves the internaliza-
                     tion of characteristics of the object with the goal of close-
                     ness to and constant presence of the object. Anxiety con-
                     sequent to separation or tension arising out of ambivalence
                     toward the object is thus diminished. If the object is a lost
                     object, introjection nullifies or negates the loss by taking on
                     characteristics of the object, thus in a sense internally pre-
                     serving the object. Even if the object is not lost, the inter-
                     nalization usually involves a shift of cathexis reflecting a
                     significant alteration in the object relationships. Introjec-
                     tion of a feared object serves to avoid anxiety through in-
                     ternalizing the aggressive characteristic of the object, and
                     thereby putting the aggression under one's own control. The
                     aggression is no longer felt as coming from outside, but
                     is taken within and utilized defensively, thus turning the
                     subject's weak, passive position into an active, strong one.
                     The classic example is identification with the aggressor.
                     Introjection can also be out of a sense of guilt in which
                     the self-punishing introject is attributable to the hostile-
                     destructive component of an ambivalent tie to an object.
                     Thus, the self-punitive qualities of the object are taken over
                     and established within one's self as a symptom or character
                     trait, which effectively represents both the destruction and
                     the preservation of the object. This is also called identifica-
                     tion with the victim.

Table B.   Classification of Defense Mechanisms (*cont.*)

Immature Defenses (cont.)

Passive-Aggressive Behavior	Aggression toward an object expressed indirectly and ineffectively through passivity, masochism, and turning against the self.
Projection	Attributing one's own unacknowledged feelings to others; it includes severe prejudice, rejection of intimacy through suspiciousness, hypervigilance to external danger, and injustice collecting. Projection operates correlatively to introjection, such that the material of the projection is derived from the internalized configuration of the introjects. At higher levels of function, projection may take the form of misattributing or misinterpreting motives, attitudes, feelings, or intentions of others.
Regression	A return to a previous stage of development or functioning to avoid the anxieties or hostilities involved in later stages. A return to earlier points of fixation embodying modes of behavior previously given up. This is often the result of a disruption of equilibrium at a later phase of development. This reflects a basic tendency to achieve instinctual gratification or to escape instinctual tension by returning to earlier modes and levels of gratification when later and more differentiated modes fail.
Schizoid Fantasy	The tendency to use fantasy and to indulge in autistic retreat for the purpose of conflict resolution and gratification.
Somatization	The defensive conversion of psychic derivatives into bodily symptoms; tendency to react with somatic rather than psychic manifestations. Infantile somatic responses are replaced by thought and affect during development (desomatization); regression to earlier somatic forms or response (resomatization) may result from unresolved conflicts and may play an important role in psychophysiological reactions.

Neurotic Defenses

Controlling	The excessive attempt to manage or regulate events or objects in the environment in the interest of minimizing anxiety and solving internal conflicts.

Table B.   Classification of Defense Mechanisms (*cont.*)

Neurotic Defenses (cont.)

Displacement	Involves a purposeful, unconscious shifting from one object to another in the interest of solving a conflict. Although the object is changed, the instinctual nature of the impulse and its aim remain unchanged.
Dissociation	A temporary but drastic modification of character or sense of personal identity to avoid emotional distress; it includes fugue states and hysterical conversion reactions.
Externalization	A general term, correlative to internalization, referring to the tendency to perceive in the external world and in external objects components of one's own personality, including instinctual impulses, conflicts, moods, attitudes, and styles of thinking. It is a more general term than projection, which is defined by its derivation from and correlation with specific introjects.
Inhibition	The unconsciously determined limitation or renunciation of specific ego functions, singly or in combination, to avoid anxiety arising out of conflict with instinctual impulses, superego, or environmental forces or figures.
Intellectualization	The control of affects and impulses by way of thinking about them instead of experiencing them. It is a systematic excess of thinking, deprived of its affect, to defend against anxiety caused by unacceptable impulses.
Isolation	The intrapsychic splitting or separation of affect from content resulting in repression of either idea or affect or the displacement of affect to a different or substitute content.
Rationalization	A justification of attitudes, beliefs, or behavior that might otherwise be unacceptable by an incorrect application of justifying reasons or the invention of a convincing fallacy.
Reaction Formation	The management of unacceptable impulses by permitting expression of the impulse in antithetical form. This is equivalently an expression of the impulse in the negative. Where instinctual conflict is persistent, reaction formation can become a character trait on a permanent basis, usually as an aspect of obsessional character.

Table B.   Classification of Defense Mechanisms (*cont.*)

Neurotic Defenses (cont.)

Repression   Consists of the expelling and withholding from conscious awareness of an idea or feeling. It may operate either by excluding from awareness what was once experienced on a conscious level (secondary repression), or it may curb ideas and feelings before they have reached consciousness (primary repression). The "forgetting" of repression is unique in that it is often accompanied by highly symbolic behavior, which suggests that the repressed is not really forgotten. The important discrimination between repression and the more general concept of defense has been discussed.

Sexualization   The endowing of an object or function with sexual significance that it did not previously have, or possesses to a lesser degree, to ward off anxieties connected with prohibited impulses.

Mature Defenses

Altruism   The vicarious but constructive and instinctually gratifying service to others. This must be distinguished from altruistic surrender, which involves a surrender of direct gratification or of instinctual needs in favor of fulfilling the needs of others to the detriment of the self, with vicarious satisfaction only being gained through introjection.

Anticipation   The realistic anticipation of or planning for future inner discomfort: implies overly concerned planning, worrying, and anticipation of dire and dreadful possible outcomes.

Asceticism   The elimination of directly pleasurable affects attributable to an experience. The moral element is implicit in setting values on specific pleasures. Asceticism is directed against all "base" pleasures perceived consciously, and gratification is derived from the renunciation.

Humor   The overt expression of feelings without personal discomfort or immobilization and without unpleasant effect on others. Humor allows one to bear, and yet focus on, what is too terrible to be borne, in contrast to wit, which always involves distraction or displacement away from the affective issue.

Table B.   Classification of Defense Mechanisms (*cont.*)

Mature Defenses (cont.)

Sublimation	The gratification of an impulse whose goal is retained, but whose aim or object is changed from a socially objectionable one to a socially valued one. Libidinal sublimation involves a desexualization of drive impulses and the placing of a value judgment that substitutes what is valued by the superego or society. Sublimation of aggressive impulses takes place through pleasurable games and sports. Unlike neurotic defenses, sublimation allows instincts to be channeled rather than to be dammed-up or diverted. Thus, in sublimation, feelings are acknowledged, modified, and directed toward a relatively significant person or goal so that modest instinctual satisfaction results.
Suppression	The conscious or semiconscious decision to postpone attention to a conscious impulse or conflict.

References

Abraham, K. (1953). *Selected Papers on Psychoanalysis*. New York: Basic Books.

Adler, A. (1956). *The Individual Psychology of Alfred Adler* (H. L. Ansbacher and R. R. Ansbacher, eds.). New York: Basic Books.

Alexander, F. (1956). *Psychoanalysis and Psychotherapy*. New York: Norton.

Alexander, F., and Selesnick, S. T. (1966). *The History of Psychiatry*. New York: Harper & Row.

Amacher, P. (1965). *Freud's Neurological Education and Its Influence on Psychoanalytic Theory*. *Psychological Issues*, Monograph 16. New York: International Universities Press.

Balint, M. (1965). *Primary Love and Psychoanalytic Technique*. New York: Liverwright.

―――. (1968). *The Basic Fault: Therapeutic Aspects of Regression*. London: Tavistock.

Bibring, G. L., Dwyer, T. F., Huntington, D. S., and Valenstein, A. F. (1961). A study of the psychological processes in pregnancy and of the earliest mother-child relationship, II: Methodological considerations. *Psychoanalytic Study of the Child* 16:25–72

Blos, P. (1962). *On Adolescence: A Psychoanalytic Interpretation*. New York: Free Press.

Blum, H. P. (1976). Masochism, the ego ideal, and the psychology of women. *Journal of the American Psychoanalytic Association* 24 (5):157–191.

Bowlby, J. (1953). *Child Care and the Growth of Love*. Baltimore: Penguin.

―――. (1969). *Attachment and Loss*, Vol. 1, *Attachment*. New York: Basic Books.

Brenner, C. (1955). *An Elementary Textbook of Psychoanalysis*. New York: International Universities Press.

Brill, A. A. (1955). *Lectures on Psychoanalytic Psychiatry.* New York: Vintage.

Burgner, M., and Edgcumbe, R. (1972). Some problems in the conceptualization of early object-relationships, II: The concept of object constancy. *Psychoanalytic Study of the Child* 27:315–333.

Dalbiez, R. (1941). *Psychoanalytical Method and the Doctrine of Freud.* London: Longman's, Green.

Deutsch, H. (1944). *The Psychology of Women.* New York: Grune & Stratton.

———. (1965). *Neuroses and Character Types.* New York: International Universities Press.

Edgcumbe, R., and Burgner, M. (1972). Some problems in the conceptualization of early object-relationships, I: The concepts of need-satisfaction and need-satisfying relationships. *Psychoanalytic Study of the Child* 27:283–314.

Ellenberger, H. (1970). *The Discovery of the Unconscious.* New York: Basic Books.

Erikson, E. H. (1959). *Identity and the Life Cycle. Psychological Issues,* Monograph 1. New York: International Universities Press.

———. (1964). *Insight and Responsibility.* New York: Norton.

Fairbairn, W. R. D. (1954). *An Object-Relations Theory of the Personality.* New York: Basic Books.

Fenichel, O. (1945). *The Psychoanalytic Theory of Neurosis.* New York: Norton.

Ferenczi, S. (1953). *First Contributions to Psychoanalysis.* London: Hogarth.

Freud, A. (1946). *The Ego and the Mechanisms of Defense.* New York: International Universities Press.

———. (1964). *The Psychoanalytic Treatment of Children.* New York: Schocken Books.

———. (1965). *Normality and Pathology in Childhood: Assessments of Development.* New York: International Universities Press.

Freud, M. (1958). Sigmund *Freud: Man and Father.* New York: Vanguard.

Freud, S. (1953-1966). *The Standard Edition of the Complete Psychological Works of Sigmund Freud.* London: Hogarth.

———. (1954). *The Origins of Psycho-Analysis.* New York: Basic Books.

Fromm-Reichmann, F. (1950). *Principles of Intensive Psychotherapy.* Chicago: University of Chicago Press.

Gardiner, M., ed. (1971). *The Wolf Man by the Wolf Man.* New York: Basic Books.

Gill, M. M. (1963). *Topography and Systems in Psychoanalytic Theory. Psychological Issues,* Monograph 10. New York: International Universities Press.

Glover, E. (1955). *The Technique of Psychoanalysis,* 2d ed. New York: International Universities Press.

Greenacre, P. (1952). *Trauma, Growth, and Personality.* New York: International Universities Press.

Greenberg, J. R., and Mitchell, S. A. (1983). *Object Relations in Psychoanalytic Theory.* Cambridge, Mass.: Harvard University Press.

Greenson, R. (1967). *The Technique and Practice of Psychoanalysis.* New York: International Universities Press.

Guntrip, H. (1969). *Schizoid Phenomena, Object-Relations, and the Self.* New York: International Universities Press.

Hartmann, H. (1939). *Ego Psychology and the Problem of Adaptation.* New York: International Universities Press, 1958.

———. (1964). *Essays on Ego Psychology.* New York: International Universities Press.

Hartmann. H., and Kris. E. (1945). The genetic approach in psychoanalysis. *Psychoanalytic Study of the Child* 1:11–30.

Holt, R. R. (1989). *Freud Reappraised: A Fresh Look at Psychoanalytic Theory.* New York: Guilford.

Horney, K. (1939). *New Ways in Psychoanalysis.* New York: Norton.

———. (1950). *Neurosis and Human Growth.* New York: Norton.

Jacobson, E. (1964). *The Self and the Object World.* New York: International Universities Press.

Jones, E. (1953-1957). *The Life and Work of Sigmund Freud.* 3 vols. New York: Basic Books.

Jung, C. G. (1956). *Symbols of Transformation.* New York: Pantheon.

Kernberg, O. (1967). Borderline personality organization. *Journal of the American Psychoanalytic Association* 15:641–685.

———. (1970). A psychoanalytic classification of character pathology. *Journal of the American Psychoanalytic Association* 18:800–822.

Klein, M. (1932). *The Psychoanalysis of Children.* London: Hogarth.

———. (1952). *Contributions to Psychoanalysis, 1921–1945.* London: Hogarth.

———. (1957). *Envy and Gratitude.* London: Tavistock.

Kohut, H. (1966). Forms and transformations of narcissism. *Journal of the American Psychoanalytic Association* 14:243–272.

———. (1971). *The Analysis of the Self.* New York: International Universities Press.

———. (1977). *The Restoration of the Self.* New York: International Universities Press.

Kris, E. (1975). Notes on the development and on some current problems of psychoanalytic child psychology. In *Selected Papers of Ernst Kris* (L. M. Newman, ed.), pp. 54–79. New Haven: Yale University Press.

Kubie, L. S. (1950). *Practical and Theoretical Aspects of Psychoanalysis.* New York: Praeger.

Lorand, S. (1946). *Technique of Psychoanalytic Therapy.* New York: International Universities Press.

Mahler, M. S., Pine, F., and Bergmann, A. (1975). *The Psychological Birth of the Human Infant.* New York: Basic Books.

Meissner, W. W. (1977). The Wolf Man and the paranoid process. *Annual of Psychoanalysis* 5:23–74.

———. (1978). *The Paranoid Process.* New York: Aronson.

Menninger, K. A. (1958). *Theory of Psychoanalytic Technique.* New York: Basic Books.

Modell, A. H. (1968). *Object Love and Reality.* New York: International Universities Press.

Nunberg, H. (1955). *Principles of Psychoanalysis*. New York: International Universities Press.

———. (1961). *Practice and Theory of Psychoanalysis*, 2d ed. New York: International Universities Press.

Rank, O. (1958). *Beyond Psychology*. New York: Dover.

Rapaport, D. (1967). *The Collected Papers of David Rapaport* (M. M. Gill, ed.). New York: Basic Books.

Reich, W. (1949). *Character Analysis*. New York: Farrar, Straus, & Giroux.

Ricoeur, P. (1970). *Freud and Philosophy: An Essay on Interpretation*. New Haven: Yale University Press.

Rieff, P. (1961). *Freud: The Mind of the Moralist*. New York: Doubleday.

Rochlin, G. (1965). *Griefs and Discontents: The Forces of Change*. Boston: Little, Brown.

———. (1973). *Man's Aggression: The Defense of the Self*. Boston: Gambit.

Sachs, H. (1945). *Freud: Master and Friend*. Cambridge, Mass.: Harvard University Press.

Schafer, R. (1968). *Aspects of Internalization*. New York: International Universities Press.

Schur, M. (1966). *The Id and the Regulatory Principles of Mental Functioning*. New York: International Universities Press.

———. (1972). *Freud: Living and Dying*. New York: International Universities Press.

Searles, H. F. (1965). *Collected Papers on Schizophrenia and Related Subjects*. New York: International Universities Press.

Semrad, E. V. (1967). The organization of ego defenses and object loss. In *The Loss of Loved Ones* (D. M. Moriarty, ed.), pp. 126–134. Springfield, Ill.: Charles C. Thomas.

Socarides, C. W. (1974). Homosexuality. In *American Handbook of Psychiatry*, 2d ed., Vol 3 (S. Arieti, ed.), pp. 291–315. New York: Basic Books.

Spitz, R. A. (1957). *No and Yes*. New York: International Universities Press.

Spotnitz, H. (1985). *Modern Psychoanalysis of the Schizophrenic Patient*, 2d ed. New York: Human Sciences Press.

Stone, L. (1961). *The Psychoanalytic Situation*. New York: International Universities Press.

Vaillant, G. E. (1971). Theoretical hierarchy of adaptive ego mechanisms. *Archives of General Psychiatry* 24:107–118.

Waelder, R. (1960). *The Basic Theory of Psychoanalysis*. New York: International Universities Press.

Weisman, A. D. (1965). *The Existential Core of Psychoanalysis*. Boston: Little, Brown.

White, R. W. (1963). *Ego and Reality in Psychoanalytic Theory. Psychological Issues*, Monograph 11. New York: International Universities Press.

Whyte, L. L. (1962). *The Unconscious Before Freud*. Garden City, N.Y.: Doubleday.

Winnicott, D. W. (1958). *Collected Papers*. London: Tavistock.

————. (1965). *The Maturational Processes and the Facilitating Environment.* New York: International Universities Press.

Yankelovich, D., and Barrett, W. (1970). *Ego and Insight: The Psychoanalytic View of Human Nature,* rev. ed. New York: Random House.

Zetzel, E. R. (1970). *The Capacity for Emotional Growth.* New York: International Universities Press.

Zetzel, E. R., and Meissner, W. W. (1973). *Basic Concepts in Psychoanalytic Psychiatry.* New York: Basic Books.

Index

goal of, 229
as theory of therapy, 211
psychoanalytic diagnostic rationale, 212
psychoanalytic psychopathology
    about, 212–13
    borderline personality organization, 217–22
    character disorders, 213–17
    theory of neurosis, 213
    theory of psychosis, 222–24
psychoanalytic theory
    central role of narcissism, 134
    evolving concepts of self, 208–10
    life and death instincts, 141
    metapsychological assumptions, 186–91
    object relations theory, 193–202
    psychology of self, 202–4
    repressed *vs.* repressing, 70–71
    tripartite theory, 162–63
psychoanalytic treatment
    about, 234
    course of, 244–46
    free association, 234–35
    interpretation, 237–38
    resistance, 235–37
    results of, 246–47
psychoanalytic understanding
    feminine psychological development, 110–11
    fluidity, 3–4
    instincts, 74–76
psychological determinism, 63–64
psychological energies, 65
psychological processes, relationship with somatic processes, 80–81
psychological relationships, emergence of, 96–97
psychology
    early experimental approaches, 156
    as natural science, 10
psychoneurosis, 146

psychosexual development
    anal phase, 79, 251t
    focus on successive erotogenic zones, 89
    genital phase, 256t
    latency period, 254–55t
    oral phase, 88–91, 250t
    phallic phase, 79–80, 253–54t
    phases, 79–80
    urethral phase, 79, 252t
psychosis, theory of, 222–24
psychosocial crises, 122t
puberty, 111, 119–20
punishment dream, 58
pure pleasure ego, 92

quantity *(Q)*, 11–13

Rapaport, David, 156, 179, 190–91
rapid-eye-movement (REM) cycles, 45, 48
rapprochement phase, 101–2, 122t, 138, 220
rationalization, 260t
reaction formation, 260t
reality
    adaptation to, 172–73
    differentiation between internal and external, 106
    ego's relation to, 171–73
    importance of, 161–62
    infant's first recognition of, 89
    role in behavior, 157
    sense of, 172
reality principle, 138–39, 158, 160
reality testing, 172
regression, 60–61, 198–99, 230–31, 259t
Reich, Wilhelm, 205
representability, 51–52
repressed infantile drives, 49–50
repressed *vs.* repressing, 70–71
repression
    about, 261t
    achievement of, 159
    adoption of term, 157